HALF THE MOTHER,

TWICE THE LOVE

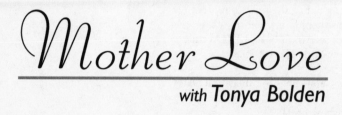

Mother Love

with Tonya Bolden

HALF THE MOTHER, TWICE THE LOVE

My Journey to Better Health with Diabetes

Resource Guide by Tamara Jeffries

ATRIA BOOKS

New York London Toronto Sydney

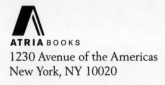
ATRIA BOOKS
1230 Avenue of the Americas
New York, NY 10020

Library of Congress Cataloging-in-Publication Data

Mother Love (Talk show host).
   Half the mother, twice the love : my journey to better health with
diabetes / Mother Love with Tonya Bolden. — 1st Atria Books trade pbk. ed.
      p. cm.
    1. Mother Love (Talk show host)—Health. 2.Diabetics—United
States—Biography. I.Bolden, Tonya. II. Title.

RC660.M62 2006
362.196'4620092—dc22
[B]
                                                                2006045889

ISBN-13: 978-0-7432-7764-8
ISBN-10:   0-7432-7764-3

First Atria Books trade paperback edition October 2006

10   9   8   7   6   5   4   3   2   1

Designed by Jaime Putorti

Manufactured in the United States of America

For information about special discounts for bulk purchases,
please contact Simon & Schuster Special Sales at
1-800-456-6798 or business@simonandschuster.com.

Smoking, pages 54–55, from: www.diabetes.org.
Copyright © 2005 American Diabetes Association.
Reprinted with permission from American Diabetes Association.

For all of my remaining family members who are struggling with diabetes and the millions of other people dealing with this disease

CONTENTS

Contents

FOREWORD

$\mathcal{I}$t is no exaggeration to say that diabetes is the epidemic of our time. In 2005 the Centers for Disease Control and Prevention (CDC) acknowledged that since 2003 the number of Americans with diabetes ballooned from 18.2 million to 20.8 million. What a sobering wake-up call this should be for each of us! Diabetes is a deadly serious disease—disrupting people's days, cutting promising lives short, stealing loved ones from us too often and too early.

Like all diseases, diabetes is an intensely personal issue, from its onset and clinical course to the impact of its complications. In this compelling book, Mother Love recounts just such a journey. We follow the course of a high-risk family, which, like so many of ours, was not sufficiently familiar with the nature of diabetes nor was the proof of prevention available at that time. We now know from clinical research that high-risk persons can prevent diabetes by following lifestyles that involve thirty or more minutes of moderate physical activity a day for at least five days each week, and a reduced-calorie, low-fat, higher-fiber diet. This approach can result in the loss of 5 percent to 7 percent of starting body weight. For a person weighing 240 pounds, this means a loss of 12 to 16 pounds over a period of one to two years! Mother Love and her family did not have the benefit of this important knowledge early on. The choices they made were, unfortunately, not the ones that would protect them from the harm that diabetes can do. There was the celebration of good cooking and heavy eating—many readers will see themselves and their families in Mother Love's family.

All of the important lessons about how we might best avoid diabetes in the first place, how to deal with it when we are affected by it, and what happens when we do not choose to take control of it are detailed in this book in ways that grip the reader and hold your interest. Mother Love makes these lessons real for us by sharing how diabetes affected real people in her life. We can feel her sense of loss as the disease strikes and disables those closest to her. We agonize with her as she seeks to overcome her life's trials by embracing her food addiction. We are inspired by her decision to take control of her diabetes. Through all of this, Mother Love does what she does so well for so many: she teaches, she shares (even some of her recipes), she challenges, and she cares.

Mother Love chose a life-changing measure to combat her obesity and thereby reduce the complications of diabetes. She is the first to admit that the route she chose is not for everyone, as she recounts the difficult emotional, social, and physical processes associated with her decision.

Being overweight or obese, having a family history of diabetes, and one's ethnicity are among the key risk factors for developing type 2 diabetes, the most common form of the disease. These are all simply predictors of who is most likely to get the disease, not guarantees of outcome. What helps determine who among those at risk will develop diabetes? The choices we make. And this is one of the most valuable lessons highlighted in Mother Love's story.

Dealing successfully with diabetes requires deciding to live life differently—making choices that promote health and peace of mind. By facing the reality of your situation and choosing to take control, you can live a healthier, more fulfilling life. This is the inspiring lesson we learn from Mother Love. Her journey with diabetes has made her who she is today and explains how she has become "half the mother" but capable of "twice the love." She has given us a real gift of enlightenment in this book. It should be read and discussed by all of us who know family members or

friends who have or who are at risk of having diabetes—
and that's a lot of us.

James R. Gavin III, MD, PhD
Executive Vice President for Clinical Affairs,
    Healing Our Village LLC
Clinical Professor of Medicine, Emory
    University School of Medicine
Past President, American Diabetes
    Association

Part One

BEFORE

Gluttony is a sin—am I going to hell?

– 1 –

GROCERY SHOPPING WAS DISNEYLAND

*M*y dad was in the kitchen at o'dark-thirty on Sunday mornings, organizing cayenne, black pepper, salt, paprika, and other spices; mincing garlic, onion, bell pepper; and cubing pork, pork fat, and beef. He was in his glory—making his signature link sausages.

If six- or seven-year-old me scrambled up and begged to help, Daddy let me add a pinch of this or that, mix the meat with my little hands, and maybe, just maybe, hold casings as he fed the meat mix into the grinder. That sausage was the centerpiece of our Sunday breakfast, likely to include grits, slab bacon, salmon croquettes, buttermilk biscuits, smothered potatoes, and fresh-squeezed OJ.

Around seven thirty, Momma had her brood heading out the door, primed to put our nickels in the offering plate and sing Jesus-loves-me hymns. In addition to me, that brood consisted of Paula, two and a half years older than me; Michael, fifteen months my junior; Fred, nineteen months younger than Michael; Marcia, eleven months younger than Fred; and Brenda, eleven months younger than Marcia.

Daddy stayed behind to clean up the kitchen and then go back to bed with Ohio's oldest black newspaper, the legendary Cleveland *Call & Post*. Whenever anyone questioned why he didn't go to church but insisted that his children attend faithfully, he said, "Well, just in case there is a GOD, I want my children to be protected."

There was no such thing as a typical Sunday dinner in our home. Each one had to be different—if not better—than the last. You wouldn't catch us having roast chicken on back-to-back Sundays. Chicken, maybe, but not prepared the same way. Momma could serve up ninety-five varieties. My favorite was what I called her "red chicken"—aka chicken cacciatore—with its sweet homemade tomato sauce graced with fresh basil and other herbs, especially garlic. We ate a lot of garlic. I don't know if Momma knew about the benefits of herbs, I just know she loved them. She also loved spices from all around the world: cinnamon from Madagascar, chilies from Mexico. She usually reserved her adventures with new spices for Sunday dinners.

Whenever we kids were introduced to a new spice or

dish from a foreign country, we had to look it up in the dictionary, find it on our globe, and read up on it in our set of encyclopedias. The kitchen was my gateway to geography. I knew where Madagascar was! My parents were avid about our education, and ours started in the kitchen. It was in the kitchen that I got my first taste of math—learning to work with measuring cups and spoons, to double or halve a recipe, and to distinguish between dry and liquid measurements.

Sunday dinner was also for putting a spin on an old standby. Instead of middle-America mashed potatoes to go with that standing rib roast, Momma might rather make garlic mashed potatoes with mushrooms and chives. OK! And they were jamming! Momma was always working her culinary skills with her blender, ricer, slicers, dicers—she even had a Kabob-It, an electric tabletop shish-kebab maker. She turned all her daughters into gadget fanatics like herself. To this day, I have to stay clear of the shopping channels, because I would own every gadget they hawk.

When holidays came around, like most American families we went into a food frenzy. We may have even out-frenzied most families, especially when it came to Thanksgiving. Three menus were the norm, finished off with a spread of sweet things to rival any bakery.

We had the traditional menu: roast turkey with oyster-and-giblet dressing; collards or a mustard-and-turnip-greens mix; macaroni and cheese casserole (longhorn and sharp cheddar aged to perfection); cranberry sauce (whole berries and jellied); and homemade cloverleaf rolls. Momma had to make dozens and dozens of rolls because over the course of the day, I could eat a dozen by myself—shoot, we all could. They were melt-in-your-mouth yumptious rolls to spread with sweet butter, sop gravy, or dip in warm honey.

Menu #2 was the "Specialty Dinner." Time to get fancy-fancy! Possibilities included roast duck, filet mignon, or a gourmet fish dish, with a couple or three side dishes, such as double-cheesy scalloped potatoes, fried-corn succotash with tomatoes and onions, or asparagus with wild mushrooms. And gravy for our veggies.

Menu #3 was the we-don't-give-a-damn-about-weight-disease-or-death menu: slow-cooked, spiced-just-right chitlins. When I researched the dish and found the correct pronunciation, I rode everybody who called them chitlins as opposed to chitterlings. To no avail. In my home, they had to be "chitlins"—fifty pounds at minimum—with hog maws mixed in. My sister Paula and brother Michael were the chitlin pickers. They sat at the sink for hours just pulling and picking poop off the hog intestines. People said that Michael "could clean a chitlin so well you could hear it squeak." I did not care who cleaned them; I refused to eat them. Everybody wanted my helping of that stinking food—always served piping hot and with hot sauce. I had no problem with the rest of the meal: spaghetti with meatballs, coleslaw, and baked or hot-water corn bread.

When my maternal great-grandmother lived with us, the hot-water corn bread was her contribution. And it took her all day to make it. She was slow-moving, and her eyesight was poor. I was her helper in the kitchen. The rest of the kids did not want to be in there with her because she was old, repeated herself, dipped snuff, chewed tobacco, and could and would spit that icky brown tobacco juice clean across the room into her spittoon. But I enjoyed her company and learned a lot from her history. She had met the self-made millionaire Madam C. J. Walker when the Madam came to the Midwest to teach "colored" women about hair care. Great-grandma also told me stories about growing up with Jim Crow in Water Valley, Mississippi, and about her migration from the South. I remember feeling so glad that I had not been born where and when she was. Not that I ever knew exactly when that was. During the few years that I knew her, Great-grandma declared herself eighty-eight, birthday after birthday.

I loved the woman, but I did not like her contribution to the Thanksgiving dinner dessert menu: molasses bread. It seemed to swell in your stomach and sit for days. And if you didn't like molasses bread, or key lime pie, or my personal favorite, German chocolate cake, you could take your pick: sweet potato pie, peach cobbler, minced meat pie, pound cake, cheesecake, cupcakes.

Preparation for Thanksgiving dinner commenced on the Monday before. All hands on deck! I was in the "low work" detail: tasks designated for the short kids. That included cleaning out the pantry, cabinets, and fridge for the new stuff coming for the celebration and getting out pots, pans, and other tools for those in the "high work" detail. They did the cutting, chopping, freezing, seasoning, and cleaning of chitlins, among other things.

As everyone did his or her part, there was laughing, singing, and sometimes fussing. Relatives and friends started coming by on that same said Monday after work to help or to just hang out. Most would bring booze; and some would bring treats for the kids. Before long, the grown-ups got a game of bid whist going. Such was our home for the next few days as we all got our mouths tuned up for the grand sit-down at two o'clock on Thursday.

We gave thanks by going back for seconds, thirds. And we always had a house full of folks. A parade of friends, kin, and pretend kin showed up to load up. Strangers, too: people a friend or relative brought along or somebody our mother adopted during the holidays. One Thanksgiving morning we woke up to find a young woman with two small boys and an infant son in our living room. OK, who were these people? Some lady who was down on her luck. Apparently, one of my cousins was the new baby's daddy. Momma felt obliged to make sure the beleaguered family at least had a happy Thanksgiving. (They stayed until right after Easter.)

After all the grown-ups had eaten to capacity, those who did not nod off were likely to be up for a "taste." A taste of Dewar's, Jack Daniel's, or Johnnie Walker Red Label. They said they needed something for the liquor to land on—the reason they ate so much, they claimed. Well, when the liquor landed, the grown-folks became really funny and our home all the louder.

When it came to Christmas dinner, as with Thanksgiving, you would have thought that we were running a restaurant. That dinner also took about a week to work up and included a standing rib roast complete with the little chef hats, which Momma made, and ornately decorated three- and four-layer cakes. For New Year's Day, we kept it simple: roast pork loin—the whole long thing—parsley potatoes, gravy, corn bread, and, of course, a monster pot of black-eyed peas for good luck. And maybe only two desserts. We could actually cook Easter dinner in one day. Typically: ham, potato salad, string beans, rolls, and only one dessert. And Kool-Aid. We had Kool-Aid with every lunch and dinner, with every snack. Kool-Aid was the first thing we children learned to make. We probably went through twenty-five pounds of sugar a week just for the Kool-Aid alone.

Whatever the meal, our parents frowned upon most all foods that came in a box or can, and anything labeled "in- stant." Just about everything we ate was fresh and made from scratch, be it for a holiday or workaday dinner—six o'clock sharp!—such as Monday's fried chicken, white rice, and salad; Tuesday's spaghetti and salad; Wednesday's beef Stroganoff and green peas; or Thursday's liver and onions with white rice, plenty of gravy, and steamed spinach. On Friday, white rice again, salad with way too much stuff in it to be healthy, and, oh, yes, here comes the fish: treated to a flour-and-cornmeal batter, then lard fried in a black cast-iron skillet. (I still have that skillet.) Most of the fish we ate had sturdy bones. We kids learned early on how to eat fish like that. Yeah, we choked sometimes, though not often.

Come Saturday morning, our family was back at the table for a big breakfast. It wasn't as big as a Sunday breakfast, but we had big bowls of cereal, lots of whole milk, and a loaf of toasted white bread. Saturday had its own happening, though: Daddy's homemade donuts. In a pot big enough to deep-fry a suckling pig, he made maybe six or seven dozen donuts for the family and for friends. He made donuts with fillings—sometimes apple butter, sometimes marmalade, jelly, or preserves. He made donuts coated with powdered sugar, drizzled with chocolate sauce, or shining with a glaze. (I swear Krispy Kreme stole my daddy's glazed donut recipe!)

As you've probably deduced by now, my family lived to eat. We loved to eat. Food was our familiar, our household god. My earliest memory of a chapter of tragic family history was the story of my father's only brother, Fred, dying a horrible death. It wasn't a head-on collision or a shark attack or a jealous husband with a switchblade. Uncle Fred, who had fallen on hard times, had starved to death. Of all the ways to exit the planet, to go out hungry was, for my family, one of the most frightening. My parents were bound and determined that would never happen to them or their children. We never went to bed hungry, never saw our cupboards bare, never wondered if we would eat another day. Food was like the sun: we knew it would come out tomorrow.

We lived lives of relative plenty in a four-bedroom cookie-cutter red-brick row-type house in Carver Park Estates—a fancy name for one of the projects in Ohio's "Mistake on the Lake," aka Cleveland. In the projects' hierarchy, we were in the upper echelon. I guess that made us upper working class. Both my parents had good jobs. Daddy was a trucker for Carling Brewery, of "Hey Mabel, Black Label!" fame. Momma worked full-time at the post office and part-time as a nurse at St. Vincent's Charity Hospital. When it came to clothes, we always had up-to-the-minute fashions and accessories. I have no memory of hand-me-downs. Our Easter outfits, custom made by Momma, were so fine that we were inevitably tapped to head up our church's Easter parade. But food, that was our pride. Food was how we celebrated ourselves. And grocery shopping was Disneyland.

On Saturdays we rose before first light, ate breakfast, piled into our gray and white Chevy something, and off we went on a long ride to get the best fruits in season and the most colorful vegetables out in the country. I remember picking strawberries from a strawberry patch and grapes off the vine. I must say, my parents did start us out on the right track when it came to fruits and vegetables. Fresh was best, they preached. Thank you, Momma and Daddy.

After we loaded up on fruits and veggies, we headed back to the city and downtown to the meat market. Paula, Michael, and I went inside to help Momma shop for the freshly ground chuck beef and pork shoulder, the bacon on a slab to be cut into the thickness we liked, and all the other meats for the week, including liver, which kids usually can't stand, but I loved.

After we stocked up on beef and pork, the next stop was the chicken market on Quincy Avenue. Daddy picked out the live chickens. We kids watched as the birds got their necks wrung, their heads chopped off, and then ran around the yard until they fell over dead. Whenever a grown-up shouted to us kids, "Sit down! Be still! You all are running around like chickens with their heads chopped off," I sat down because the visual was too much.

After the chicken market, it was on to the other stores to pick up staples, from cornmeal and flour to lard and sugar—and boring stuff like bleach, steel-wool pads, napkins, deodorant, and toilet paper.

It was a regular thing that not all the food made it home intact. We chomped into apples, we nibbled grapes. When Momma went solo into the grocery store for the staples, back in the car Daddy sometimes let the oldest kids share bottles of Carling's Black Label. Marcia and Brenda could only have sips. Between swigs of beer, we would munch on Limburger cheese and bologna off the roll, just like the old men did, crunching green onions on the side. When Momma opened the car door, she'd ball up her face like she was about to throw up through her nose. "Why do you have my kids stinking like this? This is disgusting, Joseph!" My father truly believed that beer now and then would not hurt us. Plus, I think he liked to watch our mother's reaction when she opened up the car door and almost passed out from the beer-bologna-cheese-onion funk emanating from her six kids and fat hubby. As Momma scowled, we all fell over with laughter. A lot of our laughter revolved around food. But the worst wallop I ever got from my father also had to do with food.

I was about seven and saw my father with donuts in the living room. It was a Saturday, but for some reason my father hadn't made dozens and dozens of donuts. "Oh, Daddy, can I have a donut?"

"I don't have enough for the rest of the children," he told me. "You can have this donut, but only if you eat it right here." He marked the spot with his finger.

My sibs were outside playing; Momma was tooling around in the kitchen. It was just my daddy and me in the living room. I nibbled up my donut and tucked the last chunk of it in my bottom lip when he wasn't looking. "Daddy, I'm finished. Can I go outside now?" Even I was shocked and amazed that I could speak clearly with food in my mouth.

As soon as I got on the other side of our front door, I picked that last piece of donut out of my lip and raced to taunt Paula, Michael, and Fred. "Na na na na na! Look what my daddy gave me! I got some donut, and you can't have none!"

They ran into the house with such speed that in what seemed like a second, I heard, "You little big-mouthed heifer, come here right now!" When I got within a foot of Daddy:

"Didn't I tell you not to—"

Wham! His backhand sent me sailing through the living room and into the kitchen where Momma was cooking. A wall stopped my flight. Calmly, Momma turned her head. She looked at me, then at Daddy. "Oh, your ass going to jail for hitting my baby like that," she said. She scooped me up in her arms, rushed downstairs to the car, and laid me down in the backseat. "Baby, don't move. Be still." She placed a towel over my face. We were in an emergency room within two minutes.

I looked like I had gone a few rounds with Sonny Liston. I couldn't believe my father had done this to me—my daddy, who told me repeatedly how much he loved me and who said he would do anything for me, even die for me.

When Momma and I returned home from the hospital, Daddy showed no remorse. "Maybe you'll learn not to tattle now." That's all he said to me. As for Momma, she was not one for idle threats. She had Daddy arrested. He spent maybe three days in the slammer.

I was nine when my father was arrested again, in the winter of 1963. This time it was for drunk driving, and this time he took sick while in jail. Nobody told us children what was wrong with him. All we knew was that he had been moved to the infirmary. The next thing we heard, Daddy's coming home! February 15 was the magic date.

We supercleaned and spruced up the house for his homecoming. I'm sure a big meal was planned, but I have no memory of what it was. But I do remember my sisters Marcia and Brenda, ages five and four, sitting on the bedroom floor, rolling a ball back and forth, and having the strangest conversation.

"Daddy sleepin' in his suit," said Brenda.

"I know Momma gonna be mad he sleepin' in his good suit," said Marcia. "Why won't he wake up?" The two kept rolling the ball back and forth.

Daddy never came home. A few days after his proposed release date, he lay in a casket at the House of Wills, "sleepin'" in his good blue suit, white shirt, and red tie. My father had proudly served in the army during the Korean War, and so they buried him in America's colors.

Laughter was the cause of our dad's demise, we were told. He was telling another guy in the infirmary a joke, and after Daddy hit the punch line he laughed, laughed, laughed—fell over dead from laughing so hard. So the story went.

Nobody ever said, maybe he drank too hard. Johnnie Walker Red Label was his standard.

Nobody said, maybe he answered way too much that midget bellhop's "Call for Philip Morris!" in the commercial. My father smoked at least two packs of cigarettes a day.

Nobody said that if my six-foot-tall father had not eaten so much of his homemade sausage and donuts and Momma's chitlins and lard-fried fish, maybe he would not have ended up weighing over three hundred pounds and dead at thirty-one. It was not until years later that it was pieced together why I lost my father at an early age: a diabetes-induced heart attack. I also did not know when he died that his mother was a diabetic.

Because nobody remarked on Daddy's lifestyle, nobody

thought that we should change ours. Like Daddy, Momma had smoked for years, and she kept doing so after he died. She also kept up her love affair with that riding-boot-shod, red-jacketed, monocled, striding Johnnie Walker and her Dewar's.

On the food front, we continued to eat plenty. Yet none of us was really overweight. Momma, five-foot-eight, weighed about 160 pounds. No Twiggy, but also no whale. Her children were not fat. My sister Paula was taller and larger than most kids her age, but she was not fat; she was large. I was more than not fat. I was stick skinny.

I was mocked, ridiculed, even shunned for being so thin. Everyone said I was abnormally bony. When I was about five or so, my sister Paula often told me that Momma had found me on the steps of St. Paul's Church while on her way to the L&B grocery store. She had brought me home, and Daddy let her keep me. Paula always said that I was not a real member of the family. That's why I was so bony and homely, she said.

Later, the boys in the neighborhood were the cruelest, including the one I had a crush on for the longest time. He called me Olive Oyl. He said hateful things to me like, "If you turn sideways, I could punch you in the head and thread your bony face like a needle." He "serenaded" me with "Bony Moronie, she's as skinny as a stick of macaroni." How I hated that song! When Joe Tex had that hit "Skinny Legs and All," oh, brother. "You've got your own theme song," the boys teased.

In my world, "healthy" didn't mean unclogged arteries and

no high blood pressure. Healthy meant "meat on your bones." I venture to guess that at least 40 percent of the adults in my neighborhood were overweight if not obese. People equated skinny with sick. They thought I was sick. I thought I was sick. I did not want to be sick or die from starvation like Uncle Fred. And it was my brother Fred who was the worst when it came to the teasing I got at home. He did like to ball himself up, roll across the floor, and use me as his human bowling pin.

I was also teased for taking my time at the table. I naturally ate the way I now know we are supposed to: taking small bites, chewing well, taking at least twenty minutes to eat a meal: all the better for your digestion and for enjoying the food, allowing the flavors to mingle and the aromas to mesh. But wolfing down supersized platefuls of food was my family's tradition—a tradition guaranteed to have you eating more than you should. The healthy approach is to allow your stomach time to signal "full," not gulp down the food until you feel like you're about to burst. Until I got the hang of speeding up my eating, I often lost out. One sibling or another snatched food off my plate, thinking I did not like the meal. I was rarely a "good clean-plate girl." That's what they called you when you ate all the food on your plate: a good clean-plate girl or boy.

One of our family rites of passage that revolved around food was birthdays. Twelve was the magic age when we received the privilege of choosing the dinner menu for our birthdays.

As Paula's twelfth birthday approached, she put in for her favorite: beef Stroganoff, made with lots of sour cream and loads of beef. Mine was porterhouse steak, baked potato, salad, fresh lemonade or iced tea, and German chocolate cake. For another sibling, it was spaghetti with shrimp. And always there would be an "international" dessert. That became my department when I was twelve. After I saw how fabulous my German chocolate cake was, with frosting made from scratch—like the rest of the cake—I was too ready to be Little Miss Pastry Chef.

I soon began to spread my culinary wings and try my hand at some international main dishes. I was on it! I would look through our set of encyclopedias and get inspired by a region of the world, then plan a meal. I found Asian culture especially intriguing. That's how I came to make Peking duck as part of the specialty menu for one Thanksgiving dinner. Both ducks were great, with a nice, crispy orange glaze. But I found out I needed to have had as many ducks as there were in Peking to satisfy my family. "Yeah, it's good, but it wasn't enough," was the response I got. No one had a clue that if you are going to eat something really rich or greasy—and duck is both, as is fried anything, pastries, and so much more—you should take care to eat only a small amount. Had someone tried to introduce my family to the notion of portion control, they would have viewed it as punishment and maybe slapped the messenger, too.

After my father died, food loomed even larger in our lives. Letting a kid try her hand at duck is just one example. I have often wondered if my mother was overcompensating for our being fatherless and her increased absence because she had to work more. She worked more overtime at the post office, dropped the job at the hospital, and picked up a gig at a bar. (My mother did not change jobs; she changed professions. She later went to college and became a school-teacher, then, after more study, a social worker.)

After Daddy died, Momma's schedule was wicked. After her day job, she came home to eat and change her clothes, then head to the bar, where she worked until closing. She got home about three in the morning, slept until seven, and started again the next day. We would do well if we saw her awake for more than a few minutes during the week. Grocery shopping changed as a result of her working more. There was a rise in frozen and canned foods. Whereas before, we ate home-made noodles and spaghetti, after Daddy passed, Momma started buying boxed pastas. The boxed spaghetti looked so strange to us, with all the strands so even and the same length. Momma also switched from lard to vegetable shortening. She said that vegetable shortening was better for us. Plus, it made better cookies. As I recall, the only healthy change Momma made was to switch from white bread to wheat.

When an aunt and uncle were not living with us, Paula became our chief cook. She loved food fried, barbecued, fried, and fried. Chicken, fish, potatoes, steak—whatever. The girl could throw down.

And I was getting into the habit of wolfing down my food.

— Know Your BMI —

Experts say the old height/weight charts aren't necessarily the best way to determine whether a person needs to lose or gain weight. Instead, they use as a guide *Body Mass Index (BMI),* a measure of how much fat you're packing. If you are curious about your BMI, and math is not your strong suit, you can find BMI calculators online, for example at www.cdc.gov//nccd php//dnpa//bmi.

Here's what the numbers indicate:

Weight Status	BMI
Underweight	Below 18.5
Normal	18.5–24.9
Overweight	25.0–29.9
Obese	30.0 and above
Morbidly Obese	40.0 and above

Being overweight or obese can put you at risk of contracting diabetes, but it is far from the only risk factor. There are many diabetics who have been thin their whole lives.

– 2 –

TRAUMA DRAMA

*L*osing my father was not the only trauma of my youth. When I was fourteen, in my last year of junior high school, I saw something no one should ever see: a teacher having sex with a student. One of my classmates.

It was in the spring and the school day was done when I returned to my social studies classroom to retrieve a book I had left behind. My teacher had a girl, whom I'll call Stephanie, pressed up against a wall. Her dress was up, her panties dangling on one foot. The teacher's butt was showing, his pants around his ankles. Stephanie started to cry when she and I made eye contact. The teacher turned to see what she was looking at, then kept going. I just stood there unable to move at first. I could not believe my eyes. He stared at me until he got finished. As he pulled up his pants, that's when I ran fast down the stairs to the girls' bathroom.

I splashed water on my face and began to pace, trying to calm down. Soon Stephanie was in the bathroom, too. I started crying, then she started crying.

"Are you okay?" I finally asked.

She said she was fine. She said she had wanted "to do it." I didn't believe that for a second. I told her what the teacher did was wrong—that it was statutory rape. I knew the term because the year before one of my girlfriends had gotten pregnant by a teacher. When I heard that he had been charged with "statutory rape," to the dictionary I went.

I told Stephanie that if she did not tell, I would. She begged me not to. She repeated that she was OK: "I'm fine, I'm fine." She said that if I told anyone, I would ruin everything. She had let the teacher have his way with her because he had promised to give her an A in his class. Stephanie was a beautiful girl with the body of a dancer. She was the sweet, dainty, very ladylike type; not wild and undisciplined like me. Because of the way she carried herself, I had always thought she really had it together. Clearly, sadly, she did not.

The next day, when I was in the auditorium for study hall, Mr. Teacher walked up to me, pointed to a piece of paper on the floor, and muttered angrily, "Pick up that piece of paper."

"I didn't put it there. I ain't picking it up," I replied, without giving him eye contact. *Whap!* He slapped me upside my head with a stick. Not a ruler, a stick. I had never seen him with a stick before, but I never really paid him too much attention, unlike many other girls. It seemed that every girl had a crush on him. He was big and dark. I didn't find him attractive because I was into high-yellow boys at the time.

When Mr. Teacher drew back to hit me again, I grabbed the stick, but he twisted it out of my hand. The next thing I knew, I was on the floor and he was punching me, choking me, kicking me, slapping me. He started screaming and hollering at me—"You better do what the hell I tell you to do!" Spit was coming out of his mouth, his nose was running. He looked really crazy, and I was thinking, *This is not happening to me.* I had an out-of-body experience. The real me was sitting on the lip of the stage watching a madman beating up a girl.

Pandemonium broke out. The kids started yelling for him to stop and for me to run. Some of the bigger boys finally pulled him off me. As I tried to scramble up and away, he kicked me hard in my butt, right on my tailbone. His kick sent me flying facedown. My chin broke my fall.

When I fled from the auditorium, I headed for the assistant principal's office. I was crying when I arrived. When the assistant principal saw me all bloody and banged up, a look of disdain swept over her face. I guess she figured I had been in a fight with another student because I was known to instigate fights. As I moved toward her, she snapped, "Stand on the line and wait until I'm finished." The painted line outside her door was for students waiting to see her. I was the only student there at the time.

I walked away from her office, out of the school, and through the projects—I never hit a main street or corner—to my uncle Jake and aunt Linda's house. When my uncle came to the door, he yelled for her to come. Uncle Jake, who had been on his way to work, scooped me up in his arms. He and my aunt rushed me to the emergency room.

The MDs were tending to me when my mother arrived. She made me tell her everything. And I did, from what I had seen the teacher doing to Stephanie through the chain of events that landed me in the ER. I left the hospital with a mild concussion, a sprained arm in a sling, six stitches under my chin, a black eye, a sore neck, and a cracked coccyx, and hurting all over.

The next day Momma accompanied me to school and demanded to see the assistant principal. Momma wanted to know why I had been ignored when I showed up in her office clearly injured and in pain. How could she allow a teacher to beat on a child? Where was the SOB? What was being done about this? The assistant principal summoned Mr. Teacher to her office.

He sauntered his behind in there as if it was no big deal. He glared at me as if he would beat me down again. When the assistant principal started asking him questions about hitting me, he got all defensive—said I choked him. True, I had grabbed his tie and tried to pull myself up when he was slapping me in the face, but choke him? Please.

At first, Momma was calm as Mr. Teacher ranted and raved, and called me outta my name—a job reserved for her. But then Momma went to rocking back and forth in her chair. That church-lady Holy Ghost kind of rocking. Next thing I knew—*bip! bip!*—Momma was beating the crap out of him with a hammer she'd pulled from her purse. I am talking a put-nails-in/take-nails-out claw hammer. And Momma was waling on him! He had speed knots rising all over his head, hands, arms, everywhere. The assistant principal took cover under her desk. Momma beat Mr. Teacher until she got tired. As he lay on the floor, she kicked him in the tailbone. That done, she put her hammer back in her pocketbook, slung her pocketbook over her shoulder, took me by the hand, and said, "Come on, baby, let's go."

Off we went to lunch at a new and quite fancy Chinese restaurant across town. As I looked at the menu, I wanted to taste every dish. Momma let me have some of my wish. With my good hand and still-swollen face, I tried Szechuan beef, fish with the head still on, spicy rice, and a bean curd dish. All of it was delicious. But what really made the meal memorable was that it was the first time just Momma and I had a meal out together.

As for Mr. Teacher, he threatened to press charges against Momma. Bring it on! That was her attitude. And he had better count the costs of having it come out in court that he had *schtupped* one student and beaten up another. Mr. Teacher backed down. I later heard that he lost his teaching credentials because of behavior "unbecoming a teacher." As for me, I was transferred to another junior high, to graduate with strangers. It went around my new school that I was there because I had jumped a teacher.

Because the board of ed labeled me "incorrigible," I was also put into therapy for two years: three times a week during school hours. The therapist was a kindly man with balding white hair. He had very caring, really blue eyes. I had never seen blue eyes up close like that before.

My therapist did not think that I was incorrigible. In fact, he thought I was a pretty well-adjusted young woman, very bright, with great potential. His way of helping me work through my anger included bringing me books to read aloud to him. I loved that! He also took me on mini–field trips—to museums, to a symphony, to nice restaurants. His wife sometimes joined us, bringing me some of her homemade jams and cookies.

At the time, the therapist was one of the few adult men in my life who made me feel good about myself. Another was my father's uncle John, a tall, dark man, as fine as frog hair, who worked at a funeral home. Some Saturdays he let me come to funerals and ride with him in the limo. He always called me "baby." He said it as if he would protect me with his life and never do anything to cause me harm. He was the one who had gotten me to stop sucking my thumb and my lips. Momma had tried everything to get me out of those habits, which left me with a constant ring around my mouth and knots on my thumb. Then one day Uncle John gently said, "You are too old to be sucking your thumb," and I stopped. Sometime later, he told me I was too pretty a girl to have an ugly ring around my mouth. Then and there I stopped with the lip action.

My eating habits never came up in therapy. Good ol' Blue Eyes was kind but not all that perceptive when it came to me. He never really probed about my home life. If he had, he probably would not have gotten a whole lot of details out of me because we had been raised to keep our mouths shut about what went on behind our apartment door. So the therapist never knew that after the incident with Mr. Teacher, food became a larger part of my after-school routine. Before, I would bounce in the door, phone my girlfriends, gab for hours, do my homework, eat a little dinner, then clean up the kitchen (a job I had until I went away to college). After the incident, when I got home from school, I often headed straight for the kitchen. Food became an even closer companion after I witnessed another horror a few months after the incident with Mr. Teacher.

I was on the way to the hardware store to pick up something for my mother (another hammer, maybe). As I passed one of the local rooming houses where some of the working drunks and prostitutes lived, I saw a man and woman arguing in the doorway. She was making the most noise.

"Go on, Willa Mae, I don't want to be bothered with you and your mess today," the man finally said. Those were the last words I heard from him. Willa Mae whipped out a butcher knife and plunged it into his chest. I could not move. I could not speak. I was in shock—that's what the paramedics said.

When the police arrived, I told them what I had seen. That done, I made a beeline for Porter's corner store. I bought two honey buns the size of my head. I chomped into one before I left the store. Two minutes later, I was swallowing the last bit of the second honey bun. I was feeling better. Oh, the rush of sugar!

— Sugar Is Not So Nice —

Diabetics are already spilling sugar throughout their bloodstream. They do not need to be ingesting a whole lot of sugar, especially refined sugar. For years, health professionals have been sounding the alarm that the same applies to nondiabetics because excessive sugar can rot teeth; inhibit oxygen flow; and drain the body of precious vitamins and minerals, including Bs and calcium, and thereby contribute to an impaired immune system, osteoporosis, and other ailments.

Some sources say that the average American consumes about 150 pounds of sugar annually, or about one-third of a pound a day. That's two bags of sugar in a month—just by yourself. Many experts urge Americans to cut their sugar consumption by about 50 percent. A good place to start is to give up those teaspoons of sugar in your coffee or tea and cut back on the likes of soda, ice cream, and honey buns. But you have to bear in mind that sugar abounds in all kinds of other foods, including canned fruits, meats, soups, and vegetables; boxed breakfast cereals; cold cuts; canned and bottled fruit juices; hot dogs, ketchup, mayonnaise, peanut butter, salad dressings, and various sauces, including spaghetti sauce. How can you get around that? Do more cooking from scratch in your own kitchen so that you can control the sugar content in your food and maybe cut out a lot of what you have been consuming unawares year after year. Be a smarter shopper: learn the names of added sugars. In addition to the obvious, such as honey, molasses, and *sucrose*, they include corn syrup, *dextrose*, *fructose*, *glucose*, fruit juice concentrate, high-fructose corn syrup, and *maltose*.

My midday overeating continued into my high school years. I cooked anything, as long as it was fried. My favorite was chicken wings and french fries. I could eat six wings and four potatoes. And I did so in a flash, before anyone else got home. I did not want to share.

So that Momma wouldn't miss the food, I bought my own, with the money I made from a part-time job busting suds in the school cafeteria. On my way home, I zipped to the L&B grocery store. No going to all those stores for the meat, the fish, the veggies. I did one-stop shopping. I may have spent the most money on air freshener to get rid of the cooking smells before anyone got home. Sometimes, instead of going to the L&B after school, I stopped off at Henri's, a hamburger joint with red arches. My usual meal was two cheeseburgers, fries, and a chocolate milk shake.

I never felt so good as when I was stuffing my face. Food was calming. Food did not expect anything from me. All I had to do was eat and enjoy. And I so longed to be fat. I was still sick and tired of being skinny, of being the odd one out in my family. I was looking for ways to gain weight, to fit in, to not be ridiculed. To feel good.

With reefer came another uptick in my eating. I started smoking pot to amuse my sister Paula. I could make her laugh out loud by making faces or imitating Eartha Kitt or Flip Wilson. I would get high and entertain all of our friends. Paula's friends were happy to supply the pot. I would be the entertainment, and Paula would cook (usually fried chicken and french fries). I ended up a full-blown pothead and eventually learned to make the best reefer brownies this side of anywhere. I added that to my culinary repertoire.

Even though I had started eating more, eating faster, I was still Bony Moronie. I was also Miss Defiant when it came to obeying Momma's many rules.

"You're gonna kill her! You're gonna kill her!" Paula yelled the time Momma got me down on the kitchen floor between the radiator and the door, and stomped and kicked and stomped and kicked as I coughed up blood. Momma was trying to break me of ever breaking curfew again, something I had been doing routinely.

"Oh, I am going to kill her!" Momma said calmly. And I believe she might have had Paula not pulled her off me. Paula saved my life that day.

What Momma called discipline many today call abuse, I know. Momma was definitely from the old school when it came to chastising her children. Because I was the most unruly, she made an example of me. She sometimes woke up my sibs and made them get out of their beds to see me get a beating. She wanted them to see what would happen to them if they broke curfew, stayed on the phone when she said it was time to hang up, or gave her lip, as I constantly did.

No amount of beating could tame me. The more defiant I became, the more hard-hearted my mother became toward me. When she grew tired of beating me and putting me on punishments, she grew cold. If I asked a question, I sometimes got a one-word answer; at other times, I got, "I don't want to talk to you now." There were times when I was truly sorry for something I had done, but when I offered a sincere apology, asked for her forgiveness, and moved to hug her, she'd snap, "Get away from me." "I should have flushed you down the toilet" was one of her standard lines. What's more, she could throw a look that bored through me. Worse were the times when she wouldn't even look at me.

At least my mother didn't have a problem with me when it came to staying in school. Besides, I always did well in school. (I'd had a tutor since sixth grade, when teachers told my mother I was gifted, had great potential, and should be cultivated and cultured.) When I started my first year of high school in the fall of 1969, I was taking advanced-placement classes. Because I was still holding down a part-time job, I was buying my own clothes and school supplies. As the old folks would say, I was definitely "smelling" myself. I was even more full of sashay and sass.

To my mother's caution about something or other, I often countered with, "Ain't nothing gonna happen to me— why don't you just mind your own business and take care of your other kids?" Sometimes, I just sucked my teeth. I paid for stuff like that with a backhand every now and then and many threats to knock my teeth down my throat.

When Momma said of my sorta boyfriend, "He's too old for you!" I paid her no mind. He was the kind of guy I was prone to get a crush on: older guys—guys with jobs and cars, guys who could take me out, buy me things, not be sitting around talking about "Let's get on the bus." And older guys liked me. Though fifteen, I looked and carried my 110-pound self as if I were nineteen. And I could talk more mess than a Japanese radio. I call him "sorta boyfriend" because he did not want people to know that he was jail-baiting. He was twenty-one.

On a beautiful summer early evening when I was in my bedroom getting ready for a date with Sorta Boyfriend, I heard what I thought was a car backfiring. Then I heard people running, screaming. I rushed outside, ran up the street toward the sound and the gathering crowd.

Someone in the bar down the street had shot a white guy on a motorcycle. One of the wheels of his upended motorcycle was still spinning when I arrived on the scene. He lay half on the sidewalk, half in the street, in a pool of blood. He had ridden his motorcycle into our part of town at the wrong time, a time when get-whitey sentiments were running high because of the hassling and brutality white cops routinely dished out in the community.

"Help! Somebody get help!" I screamed. My brother Michael had followed me out into the street. "Michael, go get blankets!" He raced home and back so fast.

"Don't help that white boy!" a neighbor hollered.

"This man is shot!" I pressed myself against the gaping hole in his back, trying to stop the bleeding. "Somebody, please call the ambulance! Get help!" I kept holding him. Somehow, I wedged myself under him and managed to keep the pressure on his wound and rest his head in my lap. He started coughing up blood. When it looked as if he was trying to talk, I whispered, "Don't talk."

"Where's the ambulance?!" I was hysterical, then suddenly awash with calm. Aware that I might well be the last person to be with him, I became real peaceful and nurturing.

The guy wrapped his arms around me. I don't know where he got the strength but he was holding on to me for dear life. He gave me a look that said, Please, don't let me be by myself. "I'm right here with you, baby, I'm right here," I whispered. "I'm right here. Shhh, it's all right."

By the time the ambulance arrived about twenty minutes

later, the guy had been dead about fifteen minutes. They had to pry me off him.

"Y'all let him die!" I screamed as I pushed my way through the crowd. "Y'all just stood there! How could you be so hateful? What did he do to any of you?!"

"He was a honky!" some idiot said.

I walked home in a daze down the walkway to our house. *I will tell his momma that he was not by himself when he died, that I had stayed with him until the ambulance came.*

Seconds after I reached home, my mother came in from the store. When she saw all the blood on my brand-new hot-pink outfit, she flew into a panic—"Baby, what happened?!"—and started touching me all over, checking me for damage. "No, Momma, it's not my blood . . . a guy died in my arms." I told her what happened, how nobody wanted to help the guy. Momma was so tender toward me, so full of love.

"Momma, is it wrong to help somebody because of the color of their skin?"

"No, baby," she said as she took me to the bathroom. After she helped me clean up and change, she took my bloody pink outfit, which I never saw again.

I never made contact with the dead guy's mother. When I called the hospital, the police department, the rescue squad—"Can you tell me what his name was? Do you have his parents' address or telephone number?"—no one would give me any information.

Instead of going out with Sorta Boyfriend, I stayed home that night and ate. It was sometime after ten when I started.

It was around midnight when I left the kitchen and went to bed. The next day I was too full to eat breakfast. Instead I cleaned our entire apartment. I did everybody's housework. I had to stay busy. I had to move. I had to feel alive. And I later had a ferocious appetite.

The only time I felt good was when I was eating something. Every time I flashed back to the guy dying in my lap, every time I replayed my daddy slapping me and going to jail or heard that brain tape recorder over and over of the boys mercilessly haranguing me about how bony I was, or thought about Mr. Teacher, Momma with the hammer, Willa Mae with the butcher knife, and Daddy dead, I ate. I was comforted. I kept eating.

- 3 -

IT'S NOT JUST A LITTLE SUGAR

ive-foot-five-inch seventeen-year-old me had hefted up to over 165 pounds by the time I entered Ohio State University in Columbus in the fall of 1971. I pitied the skinny collegians and didn't understand the big girls who wanted to be skinny. One of them was a really sweet chick from Cleveland. She was the first peer who ever told me, "I admire you." She didn't, however, admire herself. She did not like being heavyset. She left school early on in her sophomore year.

Sweet Cleveland Chick had been one of the first people to call me "Sister Love," because I was nurturing by nature and ever ready with advice. When people came to her with their problems, she referred them to me. "Oh, you need to go talk to Sister Love."

There was another beautiful plus-size lady, Faith Johnson, from Dayton, a junior when I was a freshman. Faith took me under her wing and showed me how to carry myself as a beautiful, positive big girl. She gave me makeup tips and advice on how to buy the right size bra. Her advice was to "always get measured." When it came to outfits: "never look like you're trying too hard." Funny, smart, pretty—all the fellas loved Faith. I loved Faith.

"You're a big girl, go decorate yourself pretty," was Momma's advice to her daughters. We were all "healthy" by then. The love of sports saved our brothers from blimping up. They all stayed in pretty good shape until they got out of the military.

My sisters and I were not athletic. And we had no intentions of changing our eating habits one bit even though the baby of the family, Brenda, had been diagnosed with diabetes in 1969, at age eleven. Momma had to administer her *insulin* because little sister was too scared to stick herself.

I came home from college one weekend to assist with showing Brenda how to take her insulin. Momma had decided it was past time for her to grow up. Baby girl disagreed. When we tried to get Brenda to practice on an orange, she ran, screamed, and carried on as if we were trying to kill her. When I asked her questions about how she felt, she just acted as if she was not sick. She never signaled that she wanted to be what we today call "proactive" about her disease, or more simply put, that she gave a damn. She knew she had to cut down on sweets. But Brenda wanted to eat all the candy. She wanted to drink all the Kool-Aid and sugary sodas. She also loaded up her food with salt. She refused to acknowledge that her body was compromised. She did not want to understand what diabetes meant: that something had gone terribly wrong in her body; it had stopped producing insulin, the hormone that transforms sugar and other foods into energy and, in essence, into life. She had *type 1 diabetes*, aka *juvenile diabetes*. Brenda wanted to believe that when she was no longer a juvenile, she would no longer have diabetes. Not so.

The National Diabetes Information Clearinghouse (NDIC) has provided one of the best overviews of diabetes that I've come across. It reads in part:

WHAT IS DIABETES?

Diabetes is a disorder of metabolism—the way our bodies use digested food for growth and energy. Most of the food we eat is broken down into glucose, the form of sugar in the blood. Glucose is the main source of fuel for the body.

After digestion, glucose passes into the bloodstream, where it is used by cells for growth and energy. For glucose to get into cells, insulin must be present. Insulin is a hormone produced by the pancreas, a large gland behind the stomach.

When we eat, the pancreas automatically produces

the right amount of insulin to move glucose from blood into our cells. In people with diabetes, however, the pancreas either produces little or no insulin, or the cells do not respond appropriately to the insulin that is produced. Glucose builds up in the blood, overflows into the urine, and passes out of the body. Thus, the body loses its main source of fuel even though the blood contains large amounts of glucose.

WHAT ARE THE TYPES OF DIABETES?

The three main types of diabetes are

- Type 1 diabetes

- Type 2 diabetes

- Gestational diabetes

Type 1 Diabetes

Type 1 diabetes is an autoimmune disease. An autoimmune disease results when the body's system for fighting infection (the immune system) turns against a part of the body. In diabetes, the immune system attacks the insulin-producing beta cells in the pancreas and destroys them. The pancreas then produces little or no insulin. A person who has type 1 diabetes must take insulin daily to live.

At present, scientists do not know exactly what causes

the body's immune system to attack the beta cells, but they believe that autoimmune, genetic, and environmental factors, possibly viruses, are involved. Type 1 diabetes accounts for about 5 to 10 percent of diagnosed diabetes in the United States. It develops most often in children and young adults but can appear at any age.

Symptoms of type 1 diabetes usually develop over a short period, although beta-cell destruction can begin years earlier. Symptoms include increased thirst and urination, constant hunger, weight loss, blurred vision, and extreme fatigue. If not diagnosed and treated with insulin, a person with type 1 diabetes can lapse into a life-threatening diabetic coma, also known as diabetic ketoacidosis.

Type 2 Diabetes

The most common form of diabetes is type 2 diabetes. About 90 to 95 percent of people with diabetes have type 2. This form of diabetes is associated with older age, obesity, family history of diabetes, previous history of gestational diabetes, physical inactivity, and ethnicity. About 80 percent of people with type 2 diabetes are overweight.

Type 2 diabetes is increasingly being diagnosed in children and adolescents. . . .

When type 2 diabetes is diagnosed, the pancreas is usually producing enough insulin, but for unknown reasons, the body cannot use the insulin effectively, a condition called insulin resistance. After several years, insulin production decreases. The result is the same as for type 1 diabetes—glucose builds up in the blood and the body cannot make efficient use of its main source of fuel.

The symptoms of type 2 diabetes develop gradually. Their onset is not as sudden as in type 1 diabetes. Symptoms may include fatigue or nausea, frequent urination, unusual thirst, weight loss, blurred vision, frequent infections, and slow healing of wounds or sores. Some people have no symptoms.

Gestational Diabetes

Gestational diabetes develops only during pregnancy. Like type 2 diabetes, it occurs more often in African Americans, American Indians, Hispanic Americans, and among women with a family history of diabetes. Women who have had gestational diabetes have a 20 to 50 percent chance of developing type 2 diabetes within 5 to 10 years.

The National Diabetes Information Clearinghouse is a division of the National Institute of Diabetes and Digestive and Kidney Diseases (NIDDK), which is part of the U.S. Department of Health and Human Services' (HHS) National Institutes of Health (NIH). To learn more about the NDIC visit www.diabetes.niddk.nih.gov.

Though I was still a teenager when my sister was diagnosed, I wanted to learn as much as I could about diabetes—any information that would help her. There was not a lot of information out there for laypeople. It was, OK, you have diabetes: lose weight, eat right, and exercise.

I got in touch with the local chapter of the American Diabetes Association (ADA) to get a better understanding of what the organization is all about as well as to get specifics on "lose weight, eat right, and exercise." They gave me what they had at the time. When I went with Brenda to her doctor, I asked questions, too. I called pharmaceutical companies, hoping to find out about new medicines in the pipeline.

Clement Center, a neighborhood medical facility, was very helpful. I asked all kinds of questions, about everything from the symptoms of diabetes to how insulin works. I must say they were really cool, because I sometimes asked questions they could not answer. When that happened, they promised to look into it for me. As for my most pressing question, "Is there a cure?" "Not yet." I was still asking questions when I was on break from college. By then, they had tagged me "the girl with all the questions we could not answer before."

The folks at Clement appreciated my curiosity. My family, though, did not. Momma and all my sibs, including Brenda, felt that I was making too big a deal. It was "just a little sugar." Everyone has something wrong with them sometimes, they maintained. "So calm down with the questions."

By the time I went to college I knew that diabetes was

hereditary. But I never thought that could mean me, too. I kept on eating as I pleased. A damning diet was not my only bad habit. By then I had been smoking cigarettes for three years. I was the first sib to pick up that habit. Then my sister Paula started. My brand was Newport. Hers, Kool—better buzz, she said. Before long, she was hooked as well.

And there was the booze. Pagan Pink Ripple, Mad Dog 20/20, gin, then on to scotch. *Hey, I'm a woman*, I thought. I later became a Jack Daniel's devotee. As I went, so went my sibs. It seemed I was the family trendsetter.

I went about making a life for myself, always reaching for a bright future, and I found myself doing a lot of overcoming. There was the loss of two college friends in a car accident. There was the loss of another friend whose drug-induced, mind-altering experience sent him jumping from the roof of his dorm to his death. And death stalked me while home from college on summer break.

July 12, 1972.

I was at a girlfriend's house that evening, singing church songs with her and her mother when another friend joined us. My girlfriends suggested I call my Sorta Boyfriend at work (a steel mill) and have him take us for a ride in his brand-new teal blue and white Olds 98. I thought, *Why not?* I was stylin' and ready for some profilin' in a classic 1970s getup: a red, white, and blue "sizzler" outfit (a short dress with matching short-shorts) and red, white, and blue platform shoes.

Sorta Boyfriend said that he was tired but agreed to take me for a short ride. (By then, we were truly only friends.) When he picked us up, man, was I disappointed! Instead of showing up in his new car, he was in his old car. We hopped in anyway. Soon we were flying down the freeway in his 1968 Cadillac convertible.

We were about twenty minutes into our joyride, traveling about eighty-five miles an hour, when—*Bam!* The hood of the car flipped up and smashed the top of the windshield, then went back down. Sorta Boyfriend shoved me off the seat onto the floor under the dashboard. Just as he did, the hood flew back up again and unhinged, hitting him in the head. He slumped over in the passenger side, his face in front of mine. I saw one of my girlfriends grab the steering wheel from the backseat. The last thing I heard was a big thud.

I later found out that the friend who had tried to steer was hurled over an embankment. She broke her pelvis and both legs. She was in the hospital for three months. Our other friend landed in the driver's seat. The police initially thought that she was the driver because the steering wheel had broken off into her chest. She needed maybe two hundred stitches to close her body back up. Sorta Boyfriend ended up with a broken neck and collarbone. It's a wonder that anyone lived, including me.

I was balled up under the dashboard unconscious and sight unseen. The only reason they went looking for me was because they had three people to be rushed to the hospital but seven shoes. The rescue workers did the math, then started prying open the smashed-up car. They found the eighth shoe on my twisted-up foot. At the hospital, doctors did not think I would be much longer for this world—so much so that they had my shredded clothes in a bag and filled out a toe tag with my particulars. They were just waiting for a time of death.

After the doctors did their doctoring, and after my momma and her friends did their praying over me, I was wheeled out of that hospital thirty-one days later. I had survived cracked ribs, a concussion, a torn muscle in my stomach, and severe internal bleeding. I was grateful to GOD. I was humbled. And now I was convinced that I was a survivor, an overcomer. I had plans for life. Big plans. I was determined more than ever to see them through.

When I entered college, it was with a mind to major in biology. My dream was to be a mortician. (I still cherish that dream: "The Lord will bless you; Mother Love will dress you and lay you away in style!") When I returned to school after the car accident, I made no changes in my academic plan. By then I'd become comfy being called Sister Love.

And I kept up with the activism I had been engaged in since I started college. Along with protesting America's involvement in the war in Vietnam, we pressed for more tenured black and female professors, for more muscular black- and women's-studies programs, and for the creation of Hispanic studies. We also wanted university-sponsored cross-cultural events. The admins got sick of a bunch of us. In my case, they finessed a way to relieve me of my scholarship shortly before I was to start my last year of college. That was in the summer of 1974. I was bummed out but not beaten. That summer I had landed a good job with Ma Bell as an intercept operator. My plan was to keep that job, save up, and return to school for the winter quarter.

By then, I'd been with my boo for two years. I knew that Kennedy Rogers was going to be my husband the moment I spotted him stepping off an elevator in the lobby of our dorm at OSU in the fall of 1972. After I left school (and he stayed), our relationship got a lot hotter. I had my own apartment, whereas he shared one with a couple of friends. Kennedy was at my crib all the time. (He had keys and everything.) He loved my cooking, and so did his frat brothers and other friends. My apartment became the hangout.

Year by year, as thoughts of returning to school faded, I got thicker. Kennedy kept loving me along the way. And from the loving, I became pregnant in 1976. Kennedy and I hadn't planned on becoming parents, but we rolled with it. By then, we were living together.

I was "eating for two" now. I wasn't thinking that I needed to consider the nutritional needs of the life I was bringing into the world as well as my own nutritional needs. No, I was thinking I needed to eat bulk for two people. I wasn't thinking quality but, rather, quantity. So was just about everybody else in my life. Everybody wanted to feed me, and I wanted to eat with everybody. While I was fixing breakfast, I thought about what I was going to cook for dinner—maybe ribs, potato salad, German chocolate cake. My midnight snack was sharp cheddar cheese and chunks of watermelon.

When I gave birth to our son, Jahmal, on June 6, 1977, I weighed 228 pounds. Needless to say, I truly became Mother Love, and that's when I started calling myself that. Then I found out that breasts are life-sustaining mechanisms. Jahmal nursed from me like he was trying to get full and make turds. My breasts became different, like the way the rest of my body bloomed: full and large.

I had no interest in losing weight. I felt fine. I felt superbad-fine, in fact. I had a man! I had a baby! I had no idea that I was about one hundred pounds overweight. I had no concerns about my health at all. My son was my top priority. I was about doing what I had to do to provide food, shelter, and clothing for my baby and me. I was a single mother who just had to do what she had to do.

Ironically, it was motherhood and the drive to survive that led in part to my decision to try stand-up comedy. I was on a limited budget, aka welfare. No, Kennedy was not an absentee father. We had no baby momma/baby daddy drama. He just would not marry me, because he said I would not *mind* him. I would say to him, "Honey, we have sex. We are parents. I am not your child. I will not mind you!" He hated, hated, hated the fact that I was on welfare, and I hated, hated, hated that I didn't have medical insurance for our baby. That's why I went on welfare. Because Kennedy would not marry me, my son and I could not benefit from his bennies. Another irony: Kennedy worked for a major insurance company.

After I made my first money from stand-up, Kennedy was embarrassed. He said I had no business making a fool out of myself in front of people. I guess it was OK to entertain our friends and be the life of the party, but to do it and get paid, why, that was just downright unladylike.

My first shot at stand-up had come on the heels of a dare. "Since you can make me laugh out loud so hard, you could make the whole world laugh!" a friend from college had declared one day. She bet me fifty bucks that I would not take a stab at stand-up. I took the challenge.

In the late fall of 1977, I performed at open-mike night (and bikers' night!) at Oldfield's Bar and Grille in Columbus. I truly had the room on my side, and I brought down the house! If you can make bikers laugh, you are funny. The bartender flipped me twenty-five bucks and let me have all the booze I could drink. He also invited me to come back to the club.

While I did my routine, I was hungry. Afterward, I was famished. Off to the grocery store I went for the makings of my "celebration meal": porterhouse steak, french fries, salad. And Kool-Aid. This, at about one o'clock in the morning.

— Porterhouse, Oh, Porterhouse —

After years of eating beef whenever I pleased, a porterhouse steak dinner landed me in a hospital with an intestinal blockage. I swore that if I got through it, I would never have beef again. No steaks, no beef Stroganoff, no liver—not even beef broth. At the time, all I knew was that beef did not agree with me. I didn't know then that red meat generally takes longer to digest than poultry and fish, and that beef has more saturated fat ounce per ounce than chicken.

Meanwhile, diabetes was still claiming family. My paternal grandmother died of a diabetes-induced heart attack in 1978. That same year, our mother, age forty-five, was diagnosed with type 2 diabetes—aka *adult onset*. Unlike Brenda, Momma's body had not stopped producing insulin but had stopped using it efficiently. My mother didn't view the diagnosis as a wake-up call. "It's just a little sugar," she insisted.

My mother didn't think about stopping to smell the roses or engaging in any kind of self-reflection. Like most people we knew, the idea of changing her "lifestyle" was foreign to her. She didn't think she *had* a lifestyle. All she had was a life, and she felt lucky to have that. It's my sense that my mother felt that being a diabetic paled in comparison to all she had been through. She kept doing what she was doing—and then some—after she became a widow at age thirty. She survived. She kept doing what she was doing after a rear-end collision sent her through a windshield at age forty-two. After my mother was diagnosed with diabetes, her MO did not change; she kept living the way she always had. She'd have to go to the doctor a little more—shrug. She'd have to get on the needle like her daughter—shrug. It was no big deal. "It's just a little sugar." Though I've never seen any hard data linking stress and diabetes, I'm convinced that stress contributed to my mother's health problems.

Later in 1978, when my sister Paula was in her first trimester with the baby girl who would be her only child, she was diagnosed with a kind of diabetes that emerges during pregnancy. *Gestational diabetes* usually disappears after childbirth, and that's what happened with my sister. She figured she was in the clear and did nothing to change her lifestyle—kept smoking and drinking, kept overeating and not exercising. Then, about two years after she had her daughter, diabetes reared its ugly head again. In 1981 she joined the ranks of people with type 2. Doctors now know that women who get gestational diabetes are almost guaranteed to be diagnosed with type 2 diabetes later in life.

Paula took the news that she would have to take insulin shots for the rest of her life in stride. Like Brenda, like Momma, Paula was at risk for a host of problems and possibly a shorter life, but she kept rolling as if nothing had happened. "It's just a little sugar." That's what many people we knew said of diabetes. Just about every diabetic we knew seemed to know of another diabetic who ate pork rinds, smoked, and did anything else they pleased and lived as long as Methuselah.

The street name "sugar" is the worst thing that ever happened to the diabetes community. The word sounds light and innocent—sweet. The image obscures the bitter reality of this disease.

— Diabetes's Dangers —

Unmanaged or mismanaged diabetes can have devastating consequences. They include:

• Hypertension: also known as high blood pressure. The pressure on the walls of the blood vessels increases a person's chance of having a stroke and heart attack, among other things.

• Cardiovascular disease: Diabetes can negatively impact one's entire cardiovascular system; that is, the working of your heart and blood vessels. "Why people with diabetes develop cardiovascular disease earlier than people who do not have the disease is not clearly understood," states *The Joslin Guide to Diabetes*, "but studies suggest that the inflammatory process begins very early in the patient who is insulin resistant."

• Nerve damage: High blood sugar can damage nerves that relate to your limbs, leaving you with numbness in your hands, legs, or arms. Harm can also come to nerves that control other parts of the body, including the stomach, bladder, and penis. "Nearly one half of all men with diabetes develop *erectile dysfunction (ED, or impotence)*," *The Joslin Guide to Diabetes* points out. "Much less is known about how diabetes may cause specific nerve problems that affect sexual function in women," says this guide, "although it has been suggested that vaginal dryness may occur. Also, high levels of blood glucose may make women more susceptible to vaginal yeast infections, which in turn can make intercourse more painful."

• Amputations: Blood vessels can constrict and harden so that not enough blood flows down to lower limbs, and off comes a toe, foot, or leg.

• Blindness: Diabetes can wreak havoc on the retina's small blood vessels.

• Kidney disease: High blood sugar can damage your kidneys' filtering units. The damage can result in complete kidney failure.

Along with these major health risks, there are a host of "little" things that can cramp a diabetic's life, such as halitosis.

— News on Booze —

Some diabetics should not drink alcohol at all because it exacerbates ongoing problems, such as nerve damage, eye disease, and high blood pressure. Diabetics who can have alcoholic beverages must drink in moderation. "Moderation is defined as two drinks a day for men and one drink a day for women," says the ADA. "A drink is a 5-ounce glass of wine, a 12-ounce light beer, or 1½ ounces of 80-proof distilled spirits. Make sure that your medications don't require avoiding alcohol, and get your doctor's OK."

— Up in Smoke —

Smoking is hazardous to *everybody's* health—doubly, triply so for diabetics. "The best-known effect of smoking is that it causes cancer," says an ADA item under the header "Smoking Hurts Your Health." The item goes on to warn, "Smoking can also aggravate many problems that people with diabetes already face, such as heart and blood vessel disease." The ADA then offers the following eleven points of light:

• Smoking cuts the amount of oxygen reaching tissues. The decrease in oxygen can lead to a heart attack, stroke, miscarriage, or stillbirth.

• Smoking increases your cholesterol levels and the levels of some other fats in your blood, raising your risk of a heart attack.

• Smoking damages and constricts the blood vessels. This damage can worsen foot ulcers and lead to blood vessel disease and leg and foot infections.

• Smokers with diabetes are more likely to get nerve damage and kidney disease.

• Smokers get colds and respiratory infections easier.

• Smoking increases your risk for limited joint mobility.

• Smoking can cause cancer of the mouth, throat, lung, and bladder.

• People with diabetes who smoke are three times as likely to die of cardiovascular disease as are other people with diabetes.

• Smoking increases your blood pressure.

• Smoking raises your blood sugar level, making it harder to control your diabetes.

• Smoking can cause impotence.

My mother and sisters kept on smoking a lot, kept on drinking a lot of booze, and kept on eating a quality and quantity of food that contributed to their disease. My other sister, Marcia, and I did likewise. She has told me that she did not think diabetes was going to happen to her, that she would dodge that bullet. I was operating on the assumption that trouble comes in threes. Diabetes had already hit my family five times that I knew of. So wasn't I in the clear?

I actually had a patch of fitness in the early 1980s, when Kennedy and I were doing our housekeeping in Cleveland, and I was driving a school bus. I was working a split shift, and my depot was far from where we lived. Instead of spending my breaks at home eating my good cooking, I took up racquetball at a court near my depot. My body got hard, tight; I slimmed down from about size 18 to size 12. But then I was transferred to a depot down the street from my home. So long, exercise. See ya, cute body.

I had ballooned back up to a size 18/20, when Kennedy finally decided to marry me. I was on the hunt for my wedding dress and other bridal needs at a local bridal show in the winter of 1985, when life moved me onto a new path. While waiting for the bridal gown and tux fashion show to begin, a man walked out on stage to host the show. The MC was a dud. The heckles from the brides-to-be and my mother got so bad. "Oh, you are better than him on period day. He is getting on my nerves!" my mother said rather loudly. To quiet her, I decided to put us out of our misery by taking over the mike, lifting the crowd's spirits with some

Mother Love stand-up comedy. That crowd included the program manager of a local radio station, WGCL-FM, one of the bridal show's sponsors. Within a few days, I was off the bus and on the radio, answering Dear Mother Love letters in the morning, and doing sports and weather in the afternoon, with a career on the rise. I was a hit!

And I got caught up. Self-control and restraint had never been part of my MO—less so when I entered the entertainment world. I loved the attention. I was just too thrilled to dine at all the finest restaurants in the area with power moguls and celebrities when they came to town. When I did, I ordered from every menu: the wine list, the main-course menu, and the dessert menu. Along with being on the radio, I was on the road a lot doing stand-up. Being on the road meant eating whatever, whenever. And getting plenty high. Coke was ubiquitous, and so often free when hanging out with fellow entertainers. Kennedy was into the drug scene as well. We started to drift apart. Same home, separate lives—and separate drug scenes. Then, in early 1989, I was no longer a hit. WGCL was sold; so long, radio show.

I kicked up my intake of coke. I was steadily getting further and further away from my right mind. It all became painfully clear Easter week 1989, when I and a bunch of my running buddies went on a free-basing binge in a friend's home. We started on Good Friday. Early Sunday morning, I had sobered up enough to drive home. Once there, I crawled into my bed, and that was it. When I woke up, I heard *60*

Minutes going off and saw my eleven-year-old son at my bed-side. "Mommy, Mommy, we missed Easter," he said matter-of-factly.

Kennedy was at the foot of the bed. "Look, it's that white girl or us. You are getting carried away. You are out of con-trol. You've been gone two days." He didn't think *he* was out of control, however.

I swore off cocaine. Still, the next few weeks were strained. Things reached the breaking point in late April, when I got an offer to go on the road for four months. When I told Kennedy what I thought was good news, hoping he'd be happy for me, he said, "I don't care what you do." A few days before I was to go on the road, he left.

Quick, I had to scramble. What do I do with Jahmal? Momma came to the rescue, agreeing to take care of him while I was on the road, driving from town to town work-ing the clubs—Ohio, West Virginia, Indiana, Michigan, Pennsylvania. Along the way, I kept folks laughing large; I was killing them! Onstage, I did a marvelous job of mask-ing my depression. Offstage, I was lovesick, heartsick, Kennedy sick, Jahmal sick, broken-up-family sick. I was also still wincing from the loss of my radio show. I dealt with my double dose of pain and humiliation just as I had dealt with the traumas of my youth: I gorged. I ate in the car all the time. I had little choice but to do a lot of my eating in what we today call "casual dining" restaurants. I indulged myself in heavy helpings of fried chicken and french fries, or pork chops with maybe mashed potatoes on the side.

I often ordered a side order of fried chicken wings to go.

I gave myself a pat on the back for not going back to the white girl. I gave myself a pass for drinking like a fish, trading one addiction for another, on top of eating obscene amounts of food.

- *4* -

I AM OUT OF THIS TOWN

*I*n June 1989 my spirit got a boost, and my life a change of venue. A radio station in Los Angeles, KFI-AM 640, beckoned. I was soon back on the air with a four-hour nighttime call-in program. I got out of my contract for my road tour with no harsh feelings. I soon had my family back, too.

In July, after I had gotten settled in L.A., I called up Kennedy for a heart-to-heart. It was fish-or-cut-bait time. I told him that I wanted us together—wanted us to work it out—but if he truly no longer wanted to be married to me, well, then, let the divorce proceedings begin. I told him about my new gig and gave him my contact information. I told him that if we were going to work it out, it would have to be in L.A. I gave him thirty days to get it together. "Together" included his quitting drugs. Kennedy was like, "Let me think about it." The next sound he heard was *click*. He called me right back. He was in L.A. in September. A month later, Jahmal was with us. We were family again.

As I dispensed my sage, often stinging advice to my "radio babies," as I called my listeners, I became a ratings success. And Kennedy and I were working it out and both drug free.

While my life was smoothing out, my overeating got worse, and my eating schedule, atrocious. I could and often did go all day without eating. I cooked breakfast just about every morning for my husband and son, but did not partake. "I'll grab something later," I always said.

No breakfast, no lunch; I did not even hit the vending machines at work. After I signed off at one o'clock in the morning, many a night—too many nights—I thought nothing of having a huge meal. I thought I was doing something good because I always had a veggie; and if I had bread, it was whole-wheat bread. But the rest of the meal was awful. I thought nothing of frying up some fish or chicken wings at two in the morning. I washed the meal down with sweet fresh lemonade or iced tea. I longed for the lethargy that a heavy meal induces, so I could go to sleep quick and hard. Never mind the horrific nightmares I sometimes had.

— *Nighttime Is Not the Right Time* —

You should not be doing any heavy eating after dark unless you work the graveyard shift. Sleep time is when your body does repair work. When you eat a lot before going to sleep, instead of your body doing that work, it's forced to do digestive work. Unless you have an amazing metabolism, late-night eating will cause you to gain weight. When you eat dinner in the early evening, you are bound to work off some of the calories just from cleaning up the kitchen, picking up the house, and getting ready for tomorrow. When you eat heavy late at night and then go to sleep, there's no burning of calories. Rolling over in bed is not exercise.

Come January 1990, I started packing in even more food during my night feasts because I had finally had enough of poisoning my body with nicotine. I had kicked cigarettes! I had my taste buds back. My good cooking tasted better than ever. I ate more, and I felt worse. I was feeling lousy more days than not, in fact.

Then . . . I could not seem to quench my thirst.

Then . . . I was running to the bathroom every five minutes. I knew the location of every bathroom between L.A., where I worked, and Pasadena, where I lived.

Then . . . I was all the time irritable. I was snapping at

my husband and son, the neighbors, anybody and everybody.

Then . . . I began to isolate myself from friends.

I did not want to be bothered with anyone, including—and especially—my family back in Cleveland. I knew the symptoms of diabetes. Damn! I did not want their disease! When I went for my annual gynecological checkup in the spring of 1990, I had my doctor give me a *glucose tolerance test*. As I was already exhibiting symptoms I knew so well, I was certain that a glucose tolerance test was all I needed for that final answer.

My doctor called a few days later. "Well, ML, you have diabetes pretty bad. Your blood sugar is 225." At age thirty-six, I was a statistic: a type 2 diabetic. My weight matched my blood sugar: I weighed about 225 pounds. I didn't know it then, but my BMI was 37.4. I was what we now call obese.

My gynecologist referred me to an internist, who said he would start me out on pills. He prescribed *glyburide* three times a day to trigger my pancreas to secrete insulin to help my body make use of it. The doctor said that it was imperative that I change my lifestyle if I hoped to stay off insulin and keep the complications of the diabetes at bay. I would have to make some major changes in my eating habits. I would have to lose weight. I would have to exercise. To help me on my way, the doctor recommended an *endocrinologist*, a specialist in metabolic disorders.

The internist also referred me to a nutritionist. When it came to meal plans, the nutritionist's tutorial on portion control blew my mind. She balled up a fist—and it was a small fist—to indicate the size potato I should eat. She showed me a deck of cards: that was the recommended size for a piece of meat. As for veggies, she recommended one cup if raw, half a cup if cooked—but not overcooked, so they'd retain more nutrients.

I did not ever want to be on insulin! I had watched my family shoot themselves. It just didn't look like fun. So you would have thought I would have been on the case! Not so. Hey, I had already quit smoking, so wasn't I ahead of the game? Maybe. A little. But I was a long way from being out of the woods. So, yes, I took my meds. Yes, I became a "pricker"—a finger sticker. I had to get a *blood glucose meter* to test my blood sugar sometimes twelve times a day. Upon rising, I checked my fasting sugar. That's when you don't eat for twelve hours, and your blood sugar should be between 80 and 120 mg/dl (milligrams of sugar per deciliter of blood). Mine was running around 170 mg/dl when I woke up—from that night eating. And I started to buy into the lie that all I had was "just a little sugar."

— Five Blood Sugar FAQs —

- *What is blood sugar?* Blood sugar—aka blood glucose—is the by-product of your body's breakdown of carbohydrates. Blood sugar is to a body what gasoline is to a car.

• *What is the diabetic's best blood test?* The *A1C Hemo-globin test.* It determines a diabetic's overall blood sugar average. The popular analogy is that the A1C results are to a diabetic what a batting average for a season is to a baseball player. Experts differ on how many times a year a diabetic should have an A1C test. Some say at least twice a year; others say three or four times a year. Most experts maintain that for most diabetics, the target number should be under 6 percent. Armed with your A1C test results, your doctor will know if you need adjustments in your meds.

• *When should you test?* If you have type 2 diabetes, it is wise to test upon rising, two hours after you eat, and before bedtime. That's about four times per day. If you have type 1, you ought to test more often. There was a young boy on our show *dLifeTV* who tested his blood sugar twelve times a day every day! When you are active, you ought to test more often, as you are burning more calories and need more fuel.

• *Where on my body can I test?* With a variety of meters on the market, strips needing less blood, and lancets that don't feel like a needle through your fingers, testing has really gotten so much better. You can test on the fleshy part of your palm, your forearm, as well as your fingertips.

- *Is testing in public OK?* Baby, you test whenever and wherever. I test in restaurants, bathrooms, concerts, stadiums.

Please make sure to "test your blood sugar, don't guess your blood sugar."

I kept up my night eating when I landed on nighttime TV with *The Mother Love Show* in early 1991. When the show was canceled after all of six weeks, I fell into a deep depression. I had lost two radio gigs and now a TV show! (I'd been fired from KFI in late 1990.)

Food again was my solace. I ate everything on a menu except "Thank You Call Again!" I can remember making a pineapple upside-down cake and eating it all by myself. My husband didn't say a word as I ate, and ate, and ate. He just wanted me to be happy. Like me, he didn't understand my issues with food—that I was eating, eating, eating when I was down and when I was up; that I had a serious addiction to food. Kennedy loved good food, but he did not stuff himself like I did, and he never had a weight issue. Neither one of us thought about the terrible example I was setting for our son.

After a few weeks, I started to come out of my funk and isolation. I began to ask questions—lots of questions—of lay cooks, chefs, nutritionists, and diabetics who were better at managing the disease than my family had been. I wanted to know how to buy healthier foods. I wanted to know about better ways to prepare the food. I started paying closer attention to food labels, because I knew I had to know about the salt, fat, and sugar contents of a product before I put it in my mouth. I became a label-reading nut.

— Know What's in Your Food! —

Food and beverage manufacturers have to list the ingredients of their products on labels, but you are responsible for knowing what those ingredients mean for your health. Diabetics need to be aware of sodium content for the sake of their blood pressure, and sugar and fat contents for the sake of their blood sugar. And remember: carbs turn into sugar.

I finally got around to calling up my homefolks. I told them that I had their disease. I cried and cried to my mother, to my sisters. Their advice? Just go on insulin, just stop making such a big deal about "a little sugar." That was the worst advice they could have given me. But it was also a godsend. I got angry. *Oh, no, I will not stand for that! I will not be like y'all!* I thought. I was even more determined to be a "better diabetic, a smarter diabetic."

I went all-out on the offensive. I let my kitchen sink guzzle down my last gallon of Jack Daniel's. Besides, I was not getting drunk from it, and if you ain't getting drunk off Jack Daniel's, you need to stop drinking. I also swore off "the pig," thanking my Maker that I had sworn off beef years earlier. And there went the velvety seafood bisque, the "triple crown" mac and cheese (cheddar, Colby, longhorn), and a smorgasbord of other high-fat, high-salt, high-sugar, high-caloric, high-disaster dishes I had loved and lived with for years.

I made myself eat more salads. I no longer overcooked broccoli, carrots, asparagus, and other veggies till they were close to mush. I steamed. As for my fish and my chicken, not fried but baked or grilled. If I yearned for a snack, I learned to reach for fresh fruit, keeping in mind that I needed to be careful about the sugar in fresh fruit. If jonesing for something sweeter, I made it something sugar free—and found out that you have to be careful about sugar-free products. Too much can give you the runs.

I learned to eat breakfast with my family. I went to cooking seminars and health expos. I even took a nutrition class. I subscribed to magazines, read everything I could on diabetes, new technologies, new medicines being created, better treatments. I switched diabetes doctors several times in my search for one who could get my vision of a healthier life. One doctor told me I asked too many questions. He said I should just accept the fact that I have diabetes and be glad that I had a good health-care plan. You *know* I left that clown.

As I strove to be a better diabetic, I tried to get my mother and sisters Paula and Brenda to do likewise. During visits home and phone calls, I told them about all that I was learning so that they, too, could better manage the disease.

When I said, "Y'all really need to quit smoking!" I got, "Don't come in here with that former-smoker garbage— I don't want to hear it!"

When I said, "We can live better with diabetes, we can live well, we can eat better. Y'all should start a walking team," I got, "Walk your twig-and-sprig-eating ass out of here now!" What they derided as "twigs and sprigs" were fresh vegetables—especially the leafy ones—and legumes. When it came to diabetes, I was definitely not the family trendsetter. There was, however, one beautiful development in the family.

After all our years as combatants, my mother and I developed that warm-and-fuzzy mother-daughter relationship I had wanted all my life. I had matured; she had softened. We had become something like sister friends. In early August 1991, Momma visited me in L.A. for the first time. Talk about a giant step: like much of my family, my mother was travel phobic. For her to leave Cleveland was a very big deal. But she hadn't conquered her fear of flying. So her visit was truly a sojourn. Instead of a four-and-a-half-hour flight, she did a two-and-a-half-day Amtrak trip. At the time, I was back on the radio, doing a show Monday through Friday, from 10:00 p.m. to 1:00 a.m. on KLSX-FM.

During Momma's stay, we talked and laughed as we had never done before. She gave me the conversation I had longed for and had actually given up on ever hearing "the Daughter Validation Conversation," those words that make you feel that you have pleased your motherlove.

We were up in the loft of my condo, and she asked for a cool drink. As I headed downstairs to get it, she said, "Baby, I just want you to know how very proud of you I am—even though it is hard for me to wrap my brain around you being a radio talk-show host! But it suits you so well because you sure can run your mouth! You talk real pretty on the air. I can't stay up to hear your whole show because you come on too late for my body clock. I am still on Cleveland time, and that three-hour difference is working on my sleep pattern." I think for the first time in my life, I was speechless.

"I am proud of the life you have made for yourself," Momma continued. She told me that she loved my home, my husband, my son. She even loved my "slaphappy" friends, one of her many names for my gay friends. She was never rude to them, just real.

Then came the big one.

"I love you as my daughter," she said. "I am proud to be your mother. I am proud to be Mother Love's mother! So proud of you that I will call you Mother Love! You are the child I will not worry about." She asked me to take care of my sisters and brothers. Her words healed all that had ever been wrong with us. I had my motherlove!

I had recently landed my first part in a movie, Corinne the cook in *Mr. Nanny*, starring Hulk Hogan. Shooting was scheduled to start in May 1992 in Miami, Florida. I was going to surprise Momma with a trip to Florida for Mother's Day. We were going to have big fun.

But when Momma waved to me from the train station in late August 1991, I saw it in her eyes and felt it in my spirit that we would never have that big fun. And that was the last time I saw her alive. On May 5, 1992, she died suddenly of a diabetes-induced heart attack. She was two months shy of her sixtieth birthday. I miss my momma.

I know my mother could have lived longer had she taken diabetes more seriously. And she lives on in my fight for a healthier life. She lives in this book, in my strength to tell my story, my hope that it will help somebody else's motherlove avoid an early grave. Many fatherloves need to make some changes, too.

After my mother's death, I redoubled my efforts to get my sisters to stop smoking, stop drinking—or at least cut back. I redoubled my efforts to get them to bake their fish and chicken, to steam their veggies—at least once or twice a week.

"It's not just a little sugar," I told them repeatedly. Sometimes I said it gently. Sometimes I yelled. Still, they were unfazed. Even after our brother Michael suffered a fatal heart attack in 1994. For all we know, he could have had diabetes. With Michael's ripping-and-running lifestyle, getting checkups and otherwise tending to his health were the last things on his mind. He was only thirty-nine years old.

Day by day, month by month, year after year, I was faithful to the pharmaceuticals that doctors prescribed. At one point,

I was on *Glucophage* (to keep my liver from producing too much glucose) and *Actos* (to make my body more sensitive to insulin). Soon it was Glucophage and the blood-pressure med *Cozaar*—not that I had high blood pressure. (Man, was I grateful for that!) Like many drugs, Cozaar has more than one use; it can also thwart kidney disease. My taking it was a preventative measure. I was also popping an aspirin a day to keep a heart attack away.

I tried to add an exercise regimen to my daily devotions. I bought just about every piece of exercise equipment advertised on late-night TV. I had it all, from a stationary bike to the Ab Rocker. I bought everything but a Bowflex, and that was because I had no place to put it. Buying the equipment was fun and the easy part. Using it sucked. After about a week, my new toy became a clothes rack. I made every excuse, from "I don't have time," "I have a headache," and "I have cramps," to "My knees hurt." (That one was true.)

I also pinballed from diet to diet. I tried Weight Watchers and watched my weight go up because when I did not feel full, I ate more of the food. I tried Metabolife—even ended up with a gig promoting it on the radio. I lost about twenty pounds, then gained back thirty after I cut Metabolife loose because my heart beat so fast at times, I thought it was going to jump out of my chest. I also tried the vegetable-soup diet. It gave me gas so bad, I could fart a symphony. I hated the grapefruit diet because you could not put sugar on the grapefruit.

All of the diets worked. For a little while. When I went

off them and ate the food I cooked for my family, the weight came back with a vengeance because I was still overeating. Making baked or grilled chicken was a good thing. Eating four pieces of chicken at one sitting was not. I seemed to expand walking down the street. I resigned myself to buying bigger clothes.

After all the giving up, swearing off, cutting back. After all the healthier eating, healthier doing, healthier thinking. After nearly a decade, I was barely managing my disease, and so far from mastering my health. Call me Mother "Sisyphus" Love. I had failed to shake the weight. Worse, I had gained weight, exacerbating my diabetes.

That was me in my late forties. By then, I was enjoying such sweet success as the host of *Forgive or Forget*, a show tailor-made around my Mother Love personality. I was doing a matchless job of keeping up appearances. Few knew that behind the scenes, I felt as if I were dying. It was as if I could feel my organs deteriorating and my brain slowing. The weight was crushing my knees. When I walked up and down stairs, my knees would *snap, crackle,* and *pop.* My hips made a crunchy sound all their own. I weighed close to 250 pounds. If, by some miracle, I'd had an adult-onset growth spurt, 250 pounds wouldn't have been so bad. But I was still about five foot five. I had really entered deeper into the danger zone: I was morbidly obese. But I did not know what to do.

While I was on daytime TV helping people turn their lives around, solve their problems, I was in the pits. I could see no way to solve my biggest problem, a problem that was steadily making me a candidate for knee surgery, a heart attack, or some other health problem that I feared would snatch me away before I got to be a senior citizen. I felt like a failure, defeated. I was scared. I was disgusted with myself. And some nights, I could also feel a prayer: "Dear GOD, if it be your will, and I make it to fifty, I want to be fit and fabulous at fifty." By *fabulous*, I was focused on that which is not only skin-deep.

While I was on tour for my book *Forgive or Forget* in the fall of 1999, I ran into Faith Johnson, my friend from college who had tutored me on how to be a good-looking, well-dressed big girl. Faith was no longer a big girl. When I asked what motivated her to lose the weight, she simply said, "I was tired of being chubby." She became part of my inspiration to change. Thank you again, Faith Johnson.

If a supersized Mother Love had been a healthy Mother Love, I would have happily stayed big. I never ever felt that there was some skinny chick inside me longing to break free, as I've heard many women claim. I truly loved my zaftig self! But I realized I needed to let that love go if I hoped to live a better quality of life.

I want to be fit and fabulous at fifty!

Self did a lot of talking to self:

Maybe it's not just about diet?

Maybe you just haven't found the right one.

Maybe there's something screwy about my meds?

Maybe if you switch up, you'll be dead.

75

Maybe there's something else I can do to stop being sick—or, worse, dead too soon?

Maybe you should just accept the fact that you come from big people.

Maybe I can actually live past sixty-something.

Maybe you want too much.

So many maybes. Too many maybes. I was getting larger by the day.

Maybe obesity surgery?

- 5 -

A DRASTIC CHANGE IS COMING

Have you lost your last mind?" That was the gist of my husband's sentiments when I broached the subject of obesity surgery in the late 1990s. I had heard that it could help obese people with diabetes get their blood sugar under control and even off their medications. I was so excited! Not my husband. He was as opposed to obesity surgery as he had been several years prior.

In the early 1990s, a friend who weighed over 350 pounds decided to get a band put on her stomach. She needed something done. She could hardly walk without feeling as if she was going to pass out. Whenever she came over for dinner, she ate constantly. Because I made sugar-free desserts, and she was having none of that, she was always on the bring-the-dessert crew. She had such bad nutrition. She had practically raised her children in fast-food restaurants. The band would close off part of her stomach and give her a smaller pouch. Smaller pouch—no more overeating. No more overeating—weight loss. Of course, merely being smaller wouldn't make her as healthy as she could be. Unless she changed *what* she ate along with *how much* she ate, she would be in jeopardy.

I accompanied my friend to her doctor's office for her last consultation before she had the band. While in the waiting room, I asked the receptionist questions about the procedure. She happily handed me some literature, and I eagerly shared it with my husband when I reached home. You would have thought I had said, "I am leaving you!" the way he reacted.

"What's wrong with you?" my husband said. "I love you like you are. That could kill you!"

"So could this weight," I responded. All I had was a comeback at the time. I did not have the courage to pursue the matter further. By 1999 I was much more persistent because I was more afraid for myself—so scared of ending up in an early grave like my mother that I was ready to end my marriage if it came to that. Yes, I would have. I was fighting for my life at this point. I was not going to let any relationship sabotage my pursuit of better health.

This time around, I reminded my husband of a few

friends who'd had the procedure. They were still alive—and smaller.

Kennedy reminded me that I was not them; that I had an image to maintain, an image as a big girl.

I reminded him that if I didn't shed a hell of a lot of weight, I might not be *me* much longer. Image and all would be dead.

To my husband's credit, he also worried about my surviving the surgery, about possible postsurgery complications, and about the aftershocks of my trying another something— a very radical something—that was not 100 percent guaranteed to work. What would happen to me if I bet it all on obesity surgery and lost weight but then, as in times past, gained it all back—and perhaps gained more? My son, by then no Bony Moronie, also thought obesity surgery was whack.

I had seen a late-night infomercial about one particular procedure. I ordered the whole informational kit and caboodle. I begged my husband to watch the video with me. Mistake! The video made him more resistant to my having obesity surgery. "That is too much, and you are not that big!" he protested.

That became the new rant—from him, my son, and most all of my friends. "Oh, you are not that big!" I was almost 250 pounds. That was plenty big for me. I was the one lugging all the damn weight around. I was the one dreading stairs. I was the one looking at knee surgery. I was the one with the heart working harder than it should have to. I was the one on

Detrol, because what with the way diabetes can weaken your bladder (you have to pee so much), I had started to have bladder control issues. I was the one who knew I had to get extreme.

"Disgusting." "Unnecessary." "Insane." "Foolish." Everywhere I turned, that's the kind of stuff I heard. People who never had a weight problem—and some who did—came down hard on obesity surgery as some vanity act or cop-out for lazy, undisciplined slobs. I had always thought, *How brave and courageous for obese people to seize the opportunity for a chance at a better life: to walk up stairs without being in agony; to sit in a booth at a restaurant; to eat in public without eyes cutting their way, telegraphing, "Pig!"; to not have their heart explode.* I thought that could be for me.

Negative reactions to the idea of obesity surgery did not abate among family and friends.

"But you can live with diabetes!"

But how well—and for how long?

"Why do you want to do something radical like that?"

Because I have tried everything else!

Because I don't want my kidneys blowing out when I'm fifty-five—I'm just not in the mood to piss blood!

Because I don't want to lose my eyesight, develop glaucoma!

Because I have a much greater chance of having a stroke than a nondiabetic!

Because I don't want to have to have knee surgery!

Because I don't want to sit around and wait to have a heart attack!

"This is stupid. You just need more willpower."

You think I'd be willing to have my guts cut up and re-arranged if I thought something else would work? How many diets have I tried? How many pills, plans, and potions had I hung my hopes on?

I had gotten real with myself. I had faced the fact that I had an addictive personality—and that I was a food junkie. I looked back over my life and started to connect the dots: how I had been raised to view overeating as a good thing, how food became my first go-to in the face of a trauma, and how after awhile, it didn't take a trauma to trigger the overeating. It had become my way of life. I had also come to see that it was becoming my son's way of life. My epiphany really came the day I saw Jahmal doing something I'd seen him do for years but had never processed: he was eating a mile-high plate of spaghetti with my yummy tomato and turkey-sausage sauce. My spirit said, *Something's very wrong with this picture.* Seeing him, seeing myself. I started doing some soul-searching.

While I prided myself on being able to conquer some addictions through willpower alone, I realized that when it came to overeating, I needed help. I needed a powerful tool. It seemed as if no one understood that I had exhausted every remedy; that surgery was my last resort; that I, too, wondered if it would work; and that I knew it would take a hell of a lot for me to see the surgery through. Sometimes I argued with people, tried to make them put themselves in my position—asked them what alternative they advised, only to have them recommend that I use more willpower or try a diet. Well, I'd tried all of that. Sometimes I didn't bother to continue the conversation and just answered people in my head.

"We're meant to be big people."

OK, but not big sickly people. We're meant to be healthy—that's GOD's plan.

Family and friends also asked what would happen to the Regal Empress Showcase, the traveling fashion show for plus-size women I founded in 1998. "How can you promote beautiful plus-size women if you are not one of them?"

I knew I would continue to maintain that a big, beautiful woman is not an oxymoron—that was the point of my Regal Empress fashion shows. I knew I would continue to celebrate plus-size people—but not the unhealthy plus size.

Death in the OR was another possibility people were quick to bring up. Someone knew someone who flatlined during a face-lift. Someone else knew someone who went in for an appendectomy and died on the operating table because the doctors left a phone inside the body, or something else wild.

I could appreciate that some people were afraid for me, but I raged. I wanted them to be afraid of what the weight could do to me—what the weight had already done to me. I wanted them to be afraid that I might die prematurely. Almost all the negative people knew well my family history—some of them *were* my family. My sister Paula was vehemently opposed to my having weight-loss surgery. It's wrong "to let them cut on you," she said.

I was desperate for something that could help me live a better quality of life. I was ready, eager to stand up and be accountable for my decision, my life, my actions. I listened to the opinions of others. But I could not be swayed by people who really did not understand what was going on with me physically, mentally, and emotionally.

More than a few of my big-girl friends were angry with me for not being satisfied with myself. They saw my self-improvement quest as a put-down of them. As in, the more you do, the more I see how little I'm doing with myself. One girlfriend actually blurted out, "You're making me look bad—like a failure."

If this works for me, if I become a better, healthier person, how can my success make you look like a failure? If this works for me, let it be an inspiration to you. Not that you should have the surgery—for you, maybe there's another way. As the kids say: "Don't hate the player, hate the game." I'm like, don't hate, celebrate, don't let my move intimidate.

Some of the issues raised by naysayers were beneficial. People sometimes asked hard questions and posed scenarios that had never crossed my mind. It made me think, do more homework, and reality-check my commitment with a new set of what-ifs. Like, what if my insurance company wouldn't cover the surgery? I knew it would cost around thirty thousand dollars. Yes, I was ready to pay for it all out of my pocket if it came to that.

My sister Paula sounded the alarm about stitches coming undone and people ending up on death's door. I did more research on the aftercare. Yes, stitches could burst—especially if you eat whole foods too soon. I talked to a few people whose obesity surgery was two or three years behind them and who had come through successfully. They all told me that as long as I followed the post-op program to the letter, I should not have to worry about ruptured stitches. Those assurances didn't faze my sister one bit. She continued to be dead set against my having the surgery.

— Large and Not in Charge —

Being obese puts you at greater risk of contracting type 2 diabetes and other illnesses. "Obesity is associated with more than 30 medical conditions, and scientific evidence has established a strong relationship with at least 15 of those conditions," says the American Obesity Association (AOA). Its list of these conditions includes:

- Arthritis (osteoarthritis and rheumatoid arthritis)

- Cancers (among them, cancer of the breast, colon, and esophagus)

- Cardiovascular disease

- Carpal tunnel syndrome

- Deep vein thrombosis (a blood clot in a lower leg, for example)

- End stage renal disease (total or almost total kidney failure)

- Gallbladder disease

- Hypertension

- Infertility

- Liver disease

- Low back pain

- Obstetric and gynecologic complications

- Pancreatitis

- Sleep apnea

- Stroke

- Urinary stress incontinence

I continued my research on obesity surgery. I called around in state and out of state trying to find out who had the best records and best results for the surgery. I studied up on the costs, the aftercare—the whole twenty yards. Oh, this was going to be more than nine yards, I knew. I lived on the internet. I could kiss Bill Gates full on the lips for making sure I could get access to information via the web. The more I learned, the more I wanted to know. I talked to people who'd had the procedure, some who'd thought about it, others who would never do it, and many who wished they could. I knew that once I got focused, I could follow through and be a good candidate for the procedure. I knew I would succeed.

Most of my support came from people who had undergone obesity surgery. I let their stories be lessons for me, reinforcement of what to do and what not to do. Take my on-the-dessert-crew friend who had the band in the early 1990s. She refused to follow her post-op plan when it came to nutrition—refused to understand that merely being smaller is not necessarily being healthier. She continued to eat junk and before long started losing sight in one eye—and she was not a diabetic. After obesity surgery, you have to be even more vigilant and detail oriented when it comes to getting the nutrients, because you will never consume enough vitamins and minerals to keep your body functioning properly. Having obesity surgery can be a dangerous thing.

I also know a beautiful woman who had *gastric bypass surgery* in the 1970s. When I told her I was considering that obesity surgery, she said, "It could save your life. I know GOD has allowed me these past twenty-five years for a reason." I thought right then that she was there to minister to me. She had taken excellent care of herself. I decided to model myself after her. She had no regrets. I wanted none.

I knew a man who did have regrets. He had gone from 455 pounds down to about 240 pounds, and he hated the way he looked. He said he felt so much pressure to exercise because his skin was very loose. Sadly, he had not exercised as he sized down. Big mistake! When you have obesity surgery, and you start losing weight that fast and do not exercise, loose skin becomes a major problem and often requires surgery to remove and tighten.

People who have gastric bypass end up with a lot of loose skin, mostly on the belly, thighs, and upper arms. Many women get lifts for some parts of their bodies and *liposuction* for other parts. When my surgeon told me that I could start having body work done about a year after the surgery, my first thought was, *Ooh! I'm gonna get a Brazilian butt!* But that was not truly my top priority. "I just want to be healthy," I told him. "I want my blood numbers tight."

People who know little about what really goes on when you have gastric bypass think it is a quick fix. That is so not true. As drastic as the procedure sounds, the change you have to make in the way you relate to food is really the drastic part. Postsurgery success requires a lot of work. If you are not a disciplined person before the surgery, you may not do well after it. If you do not believe you will do well afterward, you should never consider it.

The more angels who entered my life to wish me well, encourage me, the more confident I became that obesity surgery was for me. One of those angels is one of my "unlikely girlfriend" friends, Linda M. She's a chichi, beautiful, successful lady who is also down-to-earth; she bases friendships on a person's essence, not on matching millions and fame. So often, when my husband and I attended one of her big Hollywood soirees, folk would kind of look at me like, "Who let *her* in?" After they saw the warm, close way Linda related to me—"Oh, Mother Love, how good to see you"—they flipped and came with the air kisses and the suck-up.

"You have to do what you have to do," said Linda M. "I will support you, pray for you, pray with you." She also let me vent.

As scared as I was about my health, I also wondered what a smaller Mother Love would mean in terms of my career. Mother Love: mountain of TLC. Mother Love: so funny, so fat, and so safe. That's the Mother Love me and millions of fans had come to know, love, and expect. People took comfort in me as "a sturdy black woman." Would I have less love if I had less fat? Would I have a problem with their having a problem with me? Would I start tripping? *Would* I be less sturdy?

"Honey, you're going to be fab whatever size you're going to be," said Linda M.

I had many conversations with GOD. "Am I messing with your masterpiece?" I asked GOD at one point. Someone at my church had told me that obesity surgery is a sin. I didn't believe it was, but it's so easy to wonder. It soon dawned on me, had I not most of my adult life been messing with GOD's temple? If GOD could forgive me for all the horrible-terrible things I'd done to my body over the years—and I truly believed He had—then how could He punish me for taking a giant step to do right by my body?

I heard GOD say: "You're no good to anybody when you are sick like that. I've got to be your primary goal, and I need you well. I need you well. Do you want to be well?"

"Lord, tell me what to do, what door to walk through."

There were bands (*vertical banded gastroplasty,* or *VBG inflatable gastric band*) and bypasses (*jejunoileal bypass,* the *biliopancreatic diversion,* the *duodenal switch, roux-en-Y gastric bypass*). There was a lot of information to absorb, but it was not hard to grasp that whatever the procedure, it was about lowering caloric intake by limiting how much food I would be able to stomach for the rest of my life—if I followed the post-op plan. You have got to exercise. You must get your nutrients, keep hydrated, and change your lifestyle. You cannot eat chili cheesesteaks and think you will not get sick. You cannot eat chocolate bar after chocolate bar and then be surprised when you end up running to the bathroom with your pouch about to burst, and somebody else ends up picking you up off a cold tile floor.

After I identified the surgeon I would entrust with my body and got my insurance company to sign off on the procedure, I had to get an all clear from a psychiatrist before I could be scheduled for surgery. I expected a lot of "do you love/hate your mother" kinds of questions, but it didn't get that deep with the psychiatrist with whom I met. Yes, we chatted about my lifestyle, stress in my life, and family history. I told him that food had always loomed so large in my life and how as a child I'd wanted to be fat. He was more focused on my ability to cope with my life-changing eating capacity. He was concerned about whether I had the discipline for the follow-through of a major life change. He asked had I ever made a drastic change in my life. I shared with him that I had stopped doing cocaine without going into rehab and quit smoking cigarettes cold turkey after twenty years as a nicotine head. His demeanor was quiet, peaceful. His questions, succinct. He listened intently, and I noticed how he watched my body language. At one point, he asked about my unique circumstances, meaning my celebrity status. I gave him one of my snappy comebacks: "Oh, I don't think of myself as a celebrity, I am just a working entertainer." He came back with, "All right, Miss Working Entertainer, what if the business or your fans will not accept your drastic weight loss? It will be drastic, and people look at thin people differently. You will take people out of their comfort zone."

I sat there and watched my twenty-five years in the entertainment industry flash before my eyes, then I said with all due conviction and determination, "If people like me because I am fat, they don't like me. They don't even know me. I am ready to make a change in my life. For me!" I saw the psychiatrist only once. I later read his report while in my physician's office. The psychiatrist had said that I was a "determined woman" who had been able to conquer other habitual behaviors on my own yet knew when I needed help with a problem. He concluded that I would make a good candidate for the procedure. He also noted that my body language projected confidence.

Joining a support group for people who'd had obesity surgery, candidates for it, and significant others was not mandatory but strongly recommended. I had attended several meetings before I received the green light from the insurance company. Because my work has me on the road a lot, my attendance at support group meetings was catch-as-catch-can. I caught as many as I could whenever I was home. At one point, when I was home for a solid two-month stretch, I went and went and went. I was going to avail myself of everything that would enable me to make it through the surgery and be a success story.

At any given time, our group might be as few as six or as many as fifteen. Some members were young adults who apparently just sat in front of the TV and ballooned to 290 pounds—or more—before their twenty-first birthday. Among the full-on adults (the oldest about fifty-five), there was a schoolteacher who had the surgery because she wanted to be a positive example for her students, along with the fact that she had been very heavy all her life, and it was getting harder for her to carry the weight and walk around with her fourth graders. Several in the group were diabetics like me. At around 250 pounds, I was the smallest. Most weighed 350 or more. A few, more than 500 pounds.

We talked about eating issues. One woman said she was so out of control that she would get up in the middle of the night to binge and purge. Some members talked about family issues—including staying away from some relatives for fear of the fat jokes. Others talked about issues with strangers—including not wanting to leave their homes for fear of the stares.

There were very uplifting stories as well. One woman, whom I'll call Laura, shared how drastically her life changed after her surgery. She had gone from 458 pounds to about 190 pounds. Then she shed her husband. In truth, he drove her away. He couldn't deal with other men being attracted to her. He couldn't deal with her new self-confidence. He was as nasty to her as he had always been. He had been used to having her under his thumb. Throughout their marriage, he had been verbally abusive to her—in front of their five children. They had watched their father ridicule, berate, and otherwise mistreat their mother for years. They had listened to her cry rivers over the years. Finally, Laura had enough of the abuse and decided to save her life. She had not told her husband anything. She did her research, had her surgery, lost her weight, got strong, and got fed up with being the target of her husband's nasty tongue.

Encouragement to leave him came from what she thought was an unlikely source: her children. Her three sons and two daughters treated her to a new wardrobe, a ticket to California, first year's rent, and a car. They wished her love. They said, "Mom, you have been so good to us and to Dad, who did not deserve a good woman like you when you were heavy, and who does not deserve to have the new you."

Laura warned us that if we were successful in our weight loss, we needed to be prepared that many people in our lives would change toward us. She explained that people would treat us differently, act differently around us. She said some people might even look at us as a threat and want to challenge our decision to have surgery. She told us that we would have to be strong and stay prayerful. The last thing we needed was to be surrounded by negative people, because it was going to take our full concentration to heal after the surgery. Laura urged us to surround ourselves with people who would help us through the transition.

I shared my stories of triumph and tragedies as well as how my husband was not on board at first, how my family back east was not supportive, and the fact that I felt like I was dying from the inside out.

I always made them laugh—though not with fat jokes. I mostly listened. Through it all, I kept reminding myself that the surgery would not be a panacea; that I had to see it as a tool, as the start—not the endpoint—of a new beginning.

By early 2003 I was ready on all fronts. Thanks to the support group, the shrink, a few supportive friends, and lots of prayer, I was ready mentally and emotionally. The two people dearest to me, my husband and my son, were no longer in opposition. "Whatever's gonna make you happy," Jahmal had said to me, and not in the sense of whatever-whatever. "I know you're going to feel better for it," he added. Once Kennedy saw our son's turnaround and realized that I was stone serious about having the surgery, he became OK with it.

After a battery of tests, including several stress tests, an echocardiogram of my heart to make sure I could tolerate the surgery, I was ready physically. I had done my due diligence vis-à-vis visits with a nutritionist (to get schooled on the postsurgery meal plan). The insurance company was on board. I was financially ready. I was also ready in terms of procedure.

Science had been on the march since my friend had obesity surgery in the 1970s and since another friend had the band in the early 1990s. I was going to have LGB—*laparoscopic gastric bypass*—which was far less invasive, reduced bleeding and infection, and promised a brief hospital stay. LGB was not risk free, however. Possible complications included blood clots, damage to my spleen, hair loss, bowel obstruction, kidney disease, peptic ulcer, stroke. And heart attack. My thought: better to die trying than to mark time on the ruinous path I was on.

"What's the difference between a woman with a big ass and a big-ass woman?"

"J.Lo is a woman with a big ass. Mother Love is a big-ass woman."

Yeah, I had seen the film *Barbershop*. How well I remember people calling me up: "Have you heard . . . ?" "Did they pay you?"

In early 2003 I was looking forward to making that movie so very dated—at least when it came to me.

– 6 –

SHE DID NOT HAVE
TO GO OUT LIKE THAT!

$\mathcal{G}$irl, they've scheduled my surgery for April nineteenth!"
It was the Ides of March 2003. I was on the phone with my
sister Paula.

"Surgery? What kind of surgery?" There was bark and
bite in her question.

"I'm gonna have the gastric bypass. It's all set, Paula—
April nineteenth. Finally I'm getting this weight—"

"You ain't having that surgery on April nineteenth."

"Yes, Paula, I am." I flashed back to one of our many battles months earlier when I tried again to get my sister to take better care of herself.

"You are somebody's grandmother; don't you want to see him grow up?"

"Yeah, but that ain't my call." By then my sister had lost sight in one eye. She had also lost sensation in her feet and lower legs.

Did my sister really want me to stay miserable—end up like her—not do all in my power to have a better chance of seeing my grandbaby grow up? My son had had a son in September 2001.

"You ain't gonna have that surgery," Paula insisted. "Not while I'm living."

"Shut up—you're gonna see me svelte and healthy!"

"You're not doing it!" Paula repeated tired objections I was so tired of hearing: "It's just a little sugar . . . Can't just be letting people cut on you . . . You might die right there on the table, girl."

"How could you not want me to be healthy, Paula? You want me to see an early grave like Momma? Like you could?"

"Oh, I might be going to an early grave, but you ain't doing that surgery."

"Paula, ever since they diagnosed me with diabetes I've been fighting, fighting, fighting. I stopped drinking, changed my eating habits—with you always mocking me when I come home with new recipes and ideas about how to eat healthier, with you always yapping about how all I eat is twigs, sprigs, sprouts, and leaves. And I'm still fat, Paula—fat and unhealthy!"

"We big people, honey. We come from big people. Momma was big, Daddy was big. We're all big! You need to stop complaining—you are still the smallest one in the group."

"My knees are about to give out on me, Paula. My back hurts all the time. Everything on me hurts!" By then I was in tears. "I thought you'd be supportive of me by now."

"I am supportive of you getting better, but you gotta come up with something else."

"I'm doing this! I'm gonna do this for me!"

"Not gonna happen. You are not gonna have that surgery and you're certainly not having it on April nineteenth—over my dead body!"

"Then you just gonna have to be dead, because I'm gonna live!"

Click.

Ever since we were young, I was always the one to give in, cry uncle, extend the olive branch. That day was no different. When I called my sister back, I got my niece instead. She had the unenviable duty of telling her "auntie mommy" (as the next generation calls me) that her mother wouldn't take my call. Next day, same thing. "Tell her I ain't talking to her!" My sister wanted me to hear that.

Normally, hardly a day went by that Paula and I didn't talk at least once. And now, one, two, three, four days passed without a word passing between us. It was brutal, cruel even. I moped around the house, unable to think straight. I burst into tears every time I glanced at one of the many pictures of my favorite sister, up on a wall or on a table or desk. Paula had always been my ace. What with the way my mother and I clashed something horrible-terrible when I was young, there'd been no mother-daughter love bond back then. Paula had filled the void. She had been the one who stood up for me, whenever Momma railed against me as her "problem" child and lashed out. Paula became keeper of my secrets, best friend. After my husband and son came around to accepting and supporting my decision, I wanted to believe there would be a domino effect. Surely Paula would come around; surely she'd put her fears aside, give me her blessing, or at least not give me such grief.

Five days passed, and still my sister and I did not speak. An awful sense of doom consumed me. I got physically ill—couldn't sleep, couldn't eat. There was no end to the tears. My husband was unable to console me, though he and our son tried everything they could think of to help me. They even started cooking.

Momma started coming to me. When she first passed away, I could see her, touch her, talk to her in my sleep state. Never had I felt her in broad daylight when I was wide awake. But now, in the daytime I could hear her clearly, smell her fragrance in and around wherever I was—the office, a store, my bathroom. Then Daddy started coming around.

I kept putting pride aside, kept calling my sister's home, and kept getting "Tell her I ain't talking to her!" She knew those words would cut me to the quick.

*   *   *

My uncle John's daughter, Tootie, had agreed to fly out from Cleveland to be with me while I recuperated from surgery. She was one of my prayer partners. She had been supportive of my decision from the start. Instead of arriving closer to April 19, Tootie showed up on April 1. We thought it was an April Fool's joke when I got her call telling me that she was at Los Angeles International Airport. When we realized that Tootie was not pulling our leg, we hurried to pick her up. We expected to haul home quite a lot of luggage because she would be staying for about six weeks. But all my cousin had was one carry-on bag. When I asked her why she only had one little bag, she said the Lord had told her that was all she would need. I did not question her relationship with the Lord.

During the ride home, I told Tootie about my falling-out with Paula and her refusal to talk to me. Tootie told me to keep trying to reach her. So when we got home, I called again.

Like before, I got my niece. As soon as she knew it was me, she said, "Auntie Mommy, something's wrong with Momma. We don't know what's wrong with her. She looks real sick. She's real black." Not black-people black, but sick black.

"Call 911, take her to the emergency room," I said, scared crazy but trying not to scare my niece. "Where is she? Can she talk?"

"She can talk."

"Let me speak to her." As I waited, I braced myself for "Tell her I ain't talking to her!" Instead, I heard:

"Hey . . ." Her voice was low, slow, strained.

"Paula? . . . What's wrong with you?"

"Oh . . . I . . . I don't feel . . . good. You know . . . just, just . . . coming down with something."

"I think you need to go to the emergency room."

"Aw, girl, I'm, I'm all right."

"You need to go to the emergency room."

"I'm a little tired is all . . . just need, you know . . . a . . . little nap."

It was around six o'clock in the evening in Cleveland. My sister's nap turned into a deep sleep that lasted well into the following day, I found out when I next called.

When my niece answered the telephone, there was no exchange of pleasantries. "Let me speak to your mother," I said. My hands had trembled as I punched the phone number.

"Auntie Mommy, I—I don't know what's up."

"What do you mean?"

"We had a really hard time waking her up. We found her on the floor. Couldn't wake her up."

"Call 911."

"She won't let us."

I told my niece to put her mother on the phone.

Paula's "Hey, girl" was weak.

"Paula, you don't sound good at all."

"You know . . . I love you so much . . . so glad we're sisters and . . . we're friends. I'm glad you always listen to me . . . They won't listen to me around here. This is it for me. I love you . . . I love you. I'm so proud of you."

"Yeah, you can be proud of me and tell me all that to my face," I said. "I don't like the way things are, and I really don't like the way you sound."

Slowly, with what seemed last breaths, Paula said, "Getting on a plane, aren't you? No need to come . . . I'm all right, I'll be all right now."

"I'm on a plane. I'll be there, I will be there, I am on my way."

I couldn't get a flight to Cleveland that night. Part of me wanted to think it was a sign that there was no need to worry. The next day, I did what many women do to slough off stress and take a deep breath: Tootie and I went shopping.

We had just stepped into the dressing room with a handful of things when my cell phone rang.

"You gotta come home right now! Paula's dead! You gotta come home right now! She's dead!"

The words, the crying, the screaming—I couldn't catch the voice, I didn't want to catch the voice.

"Who the hell is this?"

"It's me! Your sister Marcia!" My younger sister was absolutely out of control. "We couldn't wake her up! We couldn't wake her up! She's dead, she's dead!"

I don't remember saying good-bye to Marcia or pressing "off." I remember slumping to the floor as if I had been punched in the gut. I remember being curled up tight in a ball and hearing someone wailing, *"No, GOD—noooooooooooooo! Please, GOD, noooooo!"* Then I heard hurried footsteps and voices in alarm.

I remember a hand and being blind to faces, deaf to words. Next, I saw a woman who looked like me stumbling from the dressing room with my cousin on her heels. The woman was running faster than I could run, running up a wide aisle with thick, sickening air and stabbing lights, splintering stares and gasps. As her eyes locked onto those of a man's: "My sister! My sister! My Paula—they say she's dead, she's dead!"

I was in my husband's arms, screaming, "They say she's dead! Not my sister! Not my sister! My sister is not dead!" I fell to the floor. My husband pulled me to my feet. He and Tootie took me outside to the car as people watched and someone whispered, "That's Mother Love! Ohmigod, that's Mother Love!" I struggled for the strength to shout, "No! No! No! I am Paula Hart's sister!"

I felt Paula's presence across my face. I heard, "You gotta calm down. You have to calm down. I'm all right . . . I told you I would be all right. Momma's here, Daddy's here. Our grandparents. I'm all right. You have to be strong. You cannot fall apart. You gotta calm down, calm down."

I can't calm down. I gotta know what's happening.

"It is the case. I've left. And I'm OK."

True to her word from the Lord, Tootie had only needed a small bag for her L.A. stay. Like Kennedy, Jahmal, and me, she was soon on a plane for Cleveland.

*   *   *

We gave Paula a grand send-off, on April 11, 2003. There was standing room only at Cleveland's brand-new Strowder's Funeral Chapel. People likened my sister's funeral to that of a politician or celebrity. Flowers in profusion— from all across the country. More than five hundred people attended. My sister was loved. Though so careless with her own health, she had been a legendary caretaker of others. She had nurtured many, many children at her home day-care center for more than a dozen years. She had always been a neighborhood rock. If there was a need, Paula was on the spot, with food, with money, with counsel, with the threat of slapping some sense into some crackhead.

Person after person, relatives and friends, got up at the funeral to have their say about my sister. People were moved to tell how she made them feel comfortable in their own skin, how she made them believe they could do anything positive they set their minds to do. She made us believe we could fly long before R. Kelly sang it.

They sang songs of praise and worship; some sang well, others should have just talked. Many who did get up to testify about what my sister meant to them talked a little too long. The service was well into hour two when I, the last to speak, moved to the front of the funeral home.

I said the sorts of things people expect to hear at a funeral, stifling all that was really in my heart as I looked out at the sea of faces, so many of them so overweight.

I talked about how beautiful it was that so many people turned out to remember my sister.

My sister, dead from a diabetes-induced heart attack because her big ass didn't want to quit smoking, quit drinking, quit filling up her stomach with crap! She did not have to go out like that!

"And, yes, it is true my sister had a huge heart."

Now she's dead with a huge heart!

I thanked all the people who acknowledged her generosity in their spoken and written words of condolence.

And from the looks of it, a whole lot of you need to do something about your own damn lives so you don't end up dead early like my sister! She did not have to go out like that!

As I remembered Paula, at times I moved people to laughter, as I thought, *Diabetes ain't no joke!*—and at times, to tears, as I thought, *Y'all need to be crying, all right, and some of you will be doing a whole lotta crying if you don't put your big, fat child on a program to get healthier, if you don't put your big, fat self on a program, if you don't do something to change your life, get your health together!*

My sister Marcia finally showed up. I brought the service to a roar of laughter as I acknowledged her presence and the fact that she was "late." That Paula was not "late," she was dead. Marcia "late," Paula dead, Marcia "late." Laughing to keep from crying and crying anyway.

As I looked upon my sister's dead body for the last time—man, she looked great! She looked dead, but she was a good-looking corpse, especially without that big knot on her forehead. For years I'd tried to get her to get the thing checked out—*It could be cancerous!*—and removed even if it wasn't. Even offered to pay for it. But Paula did not want to be cut on. By default, it actually happened. The undertaker had removed it, no extra charge, assuming the family would be pleased. We were. Turns out, it was a fat deposit.

Her "hairness" Sevi had done Paula's braids; Marcia and I, her makeup. My son complimented me on the gorgeous navy blue dress I had picked out for her. "Ma, Auntie Paula looks so good, she could go to the club." I was steady thinking, *My sister, my friend, is dead—she did not have to go out like that!*

Back in L.A., April 14—didn't unpack, didn't eat, only climbed into bed, longing to sleep the pain away, hoping not to dream. Being awake was hell. It meant facing my new reality: life without my sister. I cried and cried so hard. It hurt so bad, emotionally and physically, to know that for the rest of my life I would be missing my sister. Missing our daily telephone talks; our signifying. Missing my constant coaxing her to get over her fear of leaving the hood and come see my L.A. life. Missing our trying to best one another at "Remember the time . . ."

– 7 –

MANAGE YOUR SUGARS, BABY

$\mathcal{T}$he mourning had me in a zombie zone. Doubts were banging at my door like I was selling crack and the police were coming. Paula had said I was not going to have the surgery. Maybe she knew best. Maybe she had been trying to save me from a fate far worse than being dangerously overweight. Besides putting a bullet in my head or killing myself some other way, I couldn't imagine what that could be. But maybe I had been trying too hard. Maybe life was too hard.

All I wanted to do was . . . nothing. But I had some events to attend, things I had promised some public-relations friends I'd do. I bowed out of some (the shaky ones); for others, I kept my word and put on a happy face. I am, after all, Mother Love: "the Nefertiti of the Needy, the Defender of the Tender."

One of those events was a Celebrate Women luncheon. The keynote speaker was a program director for an L.A. television station. She seemed a humble woman, the kind I call "Quiet Queen." Without pretense or conceit, she recounted her amazing move up the corporate ladder, stressing her reliance on hard work, stick-to-itiveness, and faith. She also shared with us that she had recently been diagnosed with diabetes. I listened up even more.

In her impassioned speech, Quiet Queen said that she had made up her mind to take control of her disease—immediately. She mentioned an L.A. doctor who played a pivotal role in her mounting triumphs over diabetes. She had already lost twenty-five pounds. I was once again pumped! I was ripped! I was ready to go!

During the meet-and-mingle phase of the luncheon, I sought out Quiet Queen and introduced myself. I told her I wanted to know more about her doctor. When she told me he was a black American, I was eager to meet him because I felt a black physician would better understand my family history, and better see our relationship with food and diabetes in the context of our culture. I figured he would find it regrettable that my family cooked up fifty pounds of chitlins for a holiday meal and never considered the consequences of that tasty dish, but he would know what I was talking about.

Two weeks after the Celebrate Women luncheon, I was

in that doctor's office. I had gotten an appointment rather quickly because I used Quiet Queen's name.

"So what can I do for you?" the doctor asked.

I shared with him what Quiet Queen had said. I gave him my family history and a snapshot of my life since I was diagnosed with diabetes. I shared with him that I had quit smoking years earlier (1990), left my hard drinking (1992), learned to eat more nutritious food (1993). I let him know how I had tried diet after diet, how I took my meds, how I had been breaking my neck to get the weight off, only to get bigger, only to be in more pain, only to get sicker. I admitted that I sometimes found myself jonesing for fried *anything*.

I told him I had been scheduled for bypass surgery after wrestling with the notion for a while, after getting dumped on by my friends and family. Then, when I was ready and feeling, "Let the chips fall where they may!" my sister had died, I fell apart, postponed my surgery, and became a ball of confusion. I confided in him that though I thought I had conquered it, angst about my career was back on the block with a vengeance.

His response was what my response had been to naysayers in my stronger moments: if I were not here, I would not have a career.

I rambled on about the band versus bypass. He reaffirmed that with the band you have to have another surgical procedure if you ever have it removed. He thought bypass also made more sense with the advent of the much less invasive laparascopic laser bypass. Before that procedure came along, people who had bypass ended up with what looked like an autopsy scar: a big ol Y, only farther down, on their abdomen. Some people were too large for *laparascopy*, but I was not.

Quiet Queen's doctor thought I had a very good chance of success—if I followed the post-op program, he stressed. "It's imperative that you do what they tell you and follow your program for the rest of your life." He went on to talk about the devastation of diabetes, with emphasis on the toll it was taking on the black community and how it would take someone/something radical to change people's hearts and minds and eradicate the disdain many people of color have for the medical profession. He said nothing about eradicating the disdain the predominantly white medical community historically had for people of color.

"You've got this disease that will most likely cost you body parts, body functions, and quite possibly kill you if you don't do something major," said the doctor.

I was getting unstuck. Angst began to dissipate and tension to fall away. Of all that he said, the true lifeline was a question no one had ever posed.

"Do you want to manage your diabetes, or do you want to eradicate it?" He said that my medications were part of the problem. "Let me tell you about those pills. They will trigger a craving for carbohydrates." I hadn't told him that I secretly considered myself a carbohydrate addict, that my cravings for fried anything included fried bread. The doctor didn't tout obesity surgery as a cure for diabetes, but he believed it would be beneficial to me and my diabetes, given my family history of obesity, diabetes, heart disease, and premature deaths. He thought that some serious weight loss could enable me to get off my meds.

"Pretty soon you're going to be fifty," the doctor said. "What do you want to do? Do you want to be healthy? If you give yourself a fighting chance, you can have some longevity."

On that early June day of 2003, I snapped out of my funk. When I got home, I couldn't call my surgeon's office fast enough to reschedule my surgery—ASAP!

My sister was fifty-one when she died. In her late forties, she had become terrified about turning fifty. She did not believe that she would make it to sixty, just as our mother had not made it to sixty.

I will not go out like that! That was my promise, my prayer. July 28, 2003, was the earliest date I could get for the surgery.

"OK, does our deal stay in place for this surgery—you know, if something happens to you on the table or afterward?" Kennedy asked on July 27, 2003.

"Yes, our deal is still in place," I replied.

The deal my husband and I have is that when one of us dies, the other has to mourn. And we mean mourn: take to the bed, wear dark glasses, cry at the photos, let the mere mention of the gone one's name send you into a weep fest, and be too grieved to eat. This behavior continues until the insurance check clears, and then it's off to Tahiti!

My husband and I laughed, and we hugged. We hugged a lot that night. He hugged me while I cooked and while I set the table. In retrospect, I think he just wanted to feel his cushy wife one last time: to love me as I was and let me know he would love me still.

Because I was not allowed to eat for at least twelve hours before my surgery, we had dinner early, around five o'clock. For my last full-plate meal, I whipped up one of my culinary masterpieces. Scrumptious and health conscious at the same time: blackened salmon salad with assorted lettuces and a brown-sugar and pecan glaze. The beverage was fresh lemonade; the dessert, mango sorbet. My son declared the meal "off the chain."

After dinner, we three engaged in some more laughing and hugging. Then my son said a prayer for me that left me in tears. He and my husband told me repeatedly how much they loved me. Kennedy said, "I love you with the love of GOD." I knew I was doing the right thing for me. I felt like a million dollars.

Later that night, my husband took a racy photograph of me. Then we made very passionate love for the last time in a sick, fat body. Early the next morning, my husband and son accompanied me to Pasadena's Huntington Memorial Hospital, where I surrendered my body to my surgeon, Dr. David Lourie, and my tomorrows to GOD.

— *Diabetes on the Rise* —

By 2003 diabetes had become the fifth-leading cause of death in America, with some 18.2 million Americans living with the disease. More than half the nation's diabetics were women, and one out of every four black women fifty-five and older had the disease. Diabetes had a hold on more than 8 percent of whites and more than 11 percent of blacks. While all diabetics are at a higher risk for kidney failure, stroke, heart attack, lower-limb amputations, and blindness, black diabetics were at a higher risk of these devastations than non-black diabetics. In 2005 the CDC reported that the number of Americans living with diabetes increased by 14 percent, up to 20.8 million. The CDC also reported that 41 million Americans had *prediabetes* and thus were at risk of contracting type 2 diabetes.

Part Two

AFTER

I will be fit and fabulous!

- 8 -

BETTER IS NOT EASY

$\mathcal{T}$he opening of the four-phase postsurgery diet plan Dr. Lourie provided said, "It will be necessary for you to follow a nutritionally complete diet designed to allow both healthy healing and recovery as well as ensure safe weight loss during the first few months after your gastric bypass."

I had read that document fifty-leven times by the time I had the surgery. "To help prevent discomfort, overstretching of the pouch, leaks or rupture at the staple lines, and complications from poor healing or malnutrition, this diet schedule must be carefully followed."

"Must, must, must"—that had to be my watchword as I

faced the actual living out of the "Four Keys to Diet after Surgery."

Key #1: Smaller Volumes

With a pouch less than an ounce, I would have to ingest no more than two ounces every half hour, with the promise of an uptick to six to eight ounces in a few weeks. For several weeks, my intake would be all liquid all the time—breakfast, lunch, and dinner. And no gulping! I'd have to sip . . . sip . . . sip. I'd have to make each two ounces last for ten minutes. There was a time when I could wolf down a six-course meal in that amount of time. When I reached the point that I could have solids: *"You must chew your food very carefully and thoroughly and eat slowly from now on to avoid damaging your pouch."* The average human stomach can stretch to the size of a football. My stomach, reduced to the size of my thumb, could stretch to about the size of half a pear. If I were going to see this thing through—all the way through—for the rest of my life, I'd have to adhere to extreme portion control: no more than the equivalent of half a sandwich per meal.

Key #2: Proper Nutrition and Calories

That meant imbibing, ever so slowly, protein shakes for several weeks. I was so glad that my friend Paula M.M. had advised me to sample various protein powders before the surgery so that I would find one I could tolerate on a daily basis. The commercials for some protein supplements are just lies! Lies, I tell you! Some of them are chalky, flavorless, and *do not* dissolve as easily as their manufacturers claim. "Oh! They are so creamy and delicious!" ads proclaim. Yeah, if you like eating paste. One brand never did dissolve into liquid. I stirred and stirred, then put the mix in my food processor for three minutes just to get the lumps out. With that nasty drink, I would have not only lost weight, I would have starved to death! I did find, finally, a chocolate-flavored one I could abide. Mixing it sometimes with nondairy milk and sometimes with water—that was the extent of my variety when it came to the protein shake.

Key #3: Plenty of Daily Fluids

For me, "plenty" was sixty-four ounces. Some of it, water; some of it, protein shake; and some of it, juice—but not sugary and otherwise adulterated juices, but, rather, pure fruit and vegetable juices. Before I went to the hospital, I brought my juicer down from one of those forsaken cabinets and cleaned it up bright. I made sure that when I came home, an assortment of fresh pineapples, oranges, and apples would be waiting for me. In the weeks to come, sometimes I made juices straight—say, just pineapple, or just orange. Sometimes I concocted blends, such as pineapple-pear, tomato-apple, and all tomato with a splash—just a tiny splash—of Tabasco sauce. I once made a V8-like juice, with radish, celery, carrot, tomato. After awhile, I had to start hiding my juices because my family began drinking them up. At night I'd make a batch to last me a week, and don't you know half of it was gone the next day.

My plan also allowed for calorie-free drinks. Rather than buy such beverages, I simply flavored my purified water with a few squeezes of a lemon. I also kept lemon-, orange-, and pineapple-flavored ice cubes on hand to break up the monotony of the sipping . . . sipping . . . sipping.

— It's Good to Be a Water Head —

Water helps health. The more hydrated we are, the easier oxygen and nutrients flow to our cells, and the better our bodies eliminate toxins. Inadequate hydration can lead to or exacerbate acne, constipation, dry skin, fatigue, headache, sinus problems, and urinary tract infections, among other things.

They say that the average person loses several cups of water a day just from breathing. Several more cups are lost through the three Ps: perspiration, peeing, and pooping. That water must be replaced. Eight ounces eight times a day is not a hard-and-fast rule for everyone, but I'm told it's not a bad guideline. You should strive to make most, if not all, of that water just plain water. Overeaters, take note: water can be an appetite suppressant. I have been told by doctors, nutritionists, and others in the diet community that when you drink water before a meal, it will make you feel full, and you will eat less.

I would also have to give up the habit of having a beverage with my meals. My nutritionist told me that it was not wise for me to eat and drink together because doing so could result in *dumping syndrome,* a trauma to my stomach that could cause diarrhea and vomiting, and damage to my new stomach. The same could happen from ingesting food or liquid too quickly.

As I understand it, it would behoove many people to stop having a beverage with meals. As we chew, our saliva glands release enzymes to aid in digestion. When we drink during a meal, we wash away those very important enzymes and cause the body to begin working in overdrive because the necessary process has been interrupted.

Key #4: Daily Vitamins and Minerals

As with my "meals," I'd have to ingest supplements ever so slowly. No popping a tablet or capsule. I'd have to do chewables to meet the daily need of folic acid, calcium, B_{12}, and so on. For some people, vitamins and minerals can be a sometimey thing—when they have a cold, are under a lot of stress, or are feeling run-down. For me, vitamins and minerals could not be a sometimey thing. They will have to be an every-single-day-of-my-life thing because I will never consume enough food to provide my body all the nutrients I need to function properly.

Phase I of my new regimen started when I was still in the hospital. I had my procedure around seven thirty in the morning. (I wanted my doctor fresh.) My husband and son were by my side when I woke up about four hours later. They had even taken photos of me asleep. (They're gonna burn in the microwave section of hell for that one.)

When I came to, I knew where I was and what I was doing there. Thankfully, I was not in a lot of pain, as is sometimes the case immediately following the procedure. I was only a little sore from the five little incisions in my belly.

About six hours after surgery, I was walking around the hospital floor. I was also getting into the groove of sip-ping . . . sipping . . . sipping two ounces of liquid every half hour. And I had to sip *still*—I had to sit down for each meal and do nothing but focus on my sipping. I was used to doing twelve things while I ate, from making a grocery list to put-ting on a wighat. Not anymore.

Phase I allowed only for clear liquids: water, chicken broth, diluted fruit juices, such as apple and cranberry—nothing with a lot of acid and sugar, like orange and tomato juice. I stayed in the hospital overnight. Not until I peed and pooped could I go home.

I was not walking on air or sunshine when I left the hospital. I felt heavier, physically and emotionally. I felt, *Oh, GOD, what if this doesn't work! What will I do?* I was a nervous wreck. My son cracked some jokes, hoping to cheer me up. I couldn't laugh. Then it hit me: the train has left the station! No turning back! This is it! I would have a new lifestyle, and I was going to ride it until the wheels fell off!

When I reached home about noon, I entered phase II of my diet plan, which would last for two weeks. My meals would consist of juices and protein shakes. First up for me was: 12:00 p.m., two ounces of H_2O. That's how I spent the first twenty minutes at home, sipping . . . sipping . . . sipping, from a shot glass–size cup. Just as I had to do in the hospital, I had to sip *still*. As half past noon neared, I got ready for lunch: 12:30 p.m., two ounces of juice. The rest of my day went as follows:

1:00 p.m., two ounces H_2O

1:30 p.m., two ounces protein shake

2:00 p.m., two ounces H_2O

2:30 p.m., ditto

3:00 p.m., ditto

3:30 p.m., two ounces protein shake

4:00 p.m., two ounces H_2O

After that, I got ready for two ounces of pineapple juice at 4:30 p.m. to be followed a half hour later with water, then, at 5:30 p.m., two ounces protein shake for dinner! Then:

6:00 p.m., two ounces H_2O

6:30 p.m., ditto

7:00 p.m., ditto

7:30 p.m., protein shake

8:00 p.m., two ounces H_2O

8:30 p.m., two ounces juice

9:00 p.m., two ounces H_2O

9:30 p.m., two ounces protein shake

10:00 p.m., two ounces H_2O

One day at a time. I told myself to take it one day at a time, like the alcoholics do. I told myself to stay prayerful—for strength, for patience. I'd also be praying for no repeat of a dream I had a few days before I had my procedure. I call it my "Henry the Eighth" dream.

I was in a banquet hall of a castle. I wasn't *at* a table, but *on* one, prone on a platter. You've seen those shots of the suckling roasted pig with the apple in its mouth? That was me in the dream. I had no apple; I had everything in my mouth at one time. I was grabbing food off other people's plates and wolfing it down as I spun around on a lazy Susan. I was guzzling drinks, spitting seeds across the room, pulling big turkey legs off plates—chomping, chomping, chomping, then throwing the bone over my shoulder and going back for more. People in the dream were shouting, "Eat it! Eat it! You will never eat again! You will never eat again!" I tell you, I woke up gagging because in my sleep I was eating so much so fast that I had started to puke. I was screaming and in a sweat. Kennedy woke up to the noise and assured me it was just a dream. He cradled me in his arms, and I drifted off to sleep. I swear I could smell food on my breath.

Rain or shine, jet lag or a head cold, no matter what all was going on in my life, my body clock has had me up a touch before seven o'clock every morning, with rare exception. The second day after my surgery was no different. Shortly after I rose, I started my monotonous eating regimen.

I could have gone drama queen, taken to my bed, and had my husband and son serve me hand and foot. No! I was not going to do that. I felt I needed to hit this challenge right out the gate. I decided to make my family one of their favorite dinners: spaghetti with a tomato sauce thick with hot Italian-style turkey sausage. On the side, a salad of mixed greens with lemon wedges, and garlic toast.

I had to do something normal. I still wanted to do my "wifing" and my mothering. When I told my husband and son that I was making them dinner, they both said, "You don't have to cook for us." But, oh, how forlorn and forsaken they looked! If they were in a cartoon, their balloons would have read, "What are we going to do?" "How will she manage?" "Food is such a big part of our lives!" Oh, how relieved they were when I insisted on making them dinner that night.

The preparation did not feel any different. I would not let it. I cooked with the same passion I always had to make them full, satisfied, and happy. Yes, I thought about how the pasta would be just right, al dente; how the flavor of the sauce, with just the right amount of Italian spices, would caress the palate; how refreshing the crisp salad would be. The aromas filled the house. I could taste it! But I knew I could not and would not do so. That's when I knew I could do whatever I had to in order to heal and get healthy—and not make myself crazy.

I had dinner ready at six o'clock sharp. And, yes, we were going to eat together. I was going to look temptation dead in the eye. So there we sat at the table, their dinner plates spaghettied up before them, salad bowls off to one side, and the garlic toast in the middle of the table. I watched my husband and son savor their flavorful, filling meal as I sipped two ounces of protein shake.

We talked about my little cups. Kennedy and Jahmal said they hoped I would be able to abide by the postsurgery plan. "I can do this!" I said. That was my mantra all through dinner. I can do this! I can do this! I can do this!

The rule at our home is I cook and the men clean up. I don't do dishes. I don't take out trash. I don't sweep, mop, or vacuum floors. Even at my heaviest, the heaviest thing I carried besides me was my purse. Still is!

After dinner, we watched some bad TV. I answered some email. I get about four hundred a day—and I love it! I even love the "junk mail." (Sift through yours—you never know what's there.)

The next day would be another day of 7:00 a.m., two ounces H_2O . . . 9:30 a.m., two ounces protein shake . . . 12:30 p.m., two ounces juice . . . 3:30 p.m., two ounces protein shake . . . 6:00 p.m., 6:30 p.m., and 7:00 p.m., two ounces H_2O, two ounces H_2O, two ounces H_2O . . . 9:30 p.m., protein shake. And for the finish at 10:00 p.m., two ounces H_2O.

I counted my blessings. What if I were a nine-to-fiver and wasn't able to take a lot of time off from work and had to work this tedious eating regimen while on the job? Such has been the case for some people, I've heard. Kudos to them.

And big ups to all the parents who raise their children well on the food front. As I contended with my strict regimen, I was overwhelmed at times with a holy envy for people who grew up in households where it was understood that merely cooking from scratch was not the same as providing nutritional meals. Where if there was rice, it was brown rice; where veggies were more often steamed, grilled, or raw; where it was understood that the best way to sabotage a salad was to drown it in preservative-laden, artificially flavored dressing; where the sauté pan was used more often than the frying pan; and where eating slowly was praised, not mocked. How fortunate are the children growing up in families where eating obscene amounts of food at one sitting is simply not allowed; where gluttony is taken seriously as one of the seven deadly sins; and where kids are not allowed to guzzle down gallons of soda and other sugar-shocked beverages week after week. The scripture says, "Raise up a child in the way he should go." Many parents take this scripture to heart. They give their children good home training. They may also give them the 411 on substance abuse. Some even talk candidly with their children about sex and sexually transmitted diseases. But when it comes to diet, many parents fail to train their children with a right relationship to food.

— Toward a Super You —

"The foods you eat every day, from the fast food you mindlessly consume to the best meals you savor in a top restaurant, are doing much more than making you fat or thin," state Steven Pratt, MD, and Kathy Matthews in "How Your Diet Is Killing You," the introduction to their book *SuperFoods Rx: Fourteen Foods That Will Change Your Life*. The foods you eat, they add, "are making the difference between the development of chronic disease and a vigorous extended life." Here are the superfoods they champion and my take on them:

• Beans: From navy beans and pinto beans to fava beans, lentils, and flageolets, beans are a high-fiber, cholesterol-lowering, cancer-fighting, low-fat food as well as a good source of protein. If you prepare dried beans instead of canned products, you spare your body unnecessary sodium. As for the flatulence factor, you may want to try some Beano, a digestive aid that can eliminate your fear of flatulence from beans as well as a host of gas-producing grains and vegetables.

• Blueberries: one of my faves when it comes to fruits— great source of manganese, vitamin K, and vitamin C, and low in cholesterol, sodium, and saturated fats.

• Broccoli: one of my favorite sprouts. Along with being a good source of fiber and protein, broccoli's blessings include many vitamins (A, B, C, E, K) and minerals (calcium, iron, magnesium, phosphorus, and potassium, among others).

• Oranges: I sometimes put oranges in the fridge, let them get cold, slice them up, and, man, what a refreshing snack!—with the bonus of vitamin C.

• Oats: You cannot beat a good bowl of oatmeal on a chilly day. OK, I can eat oatmeal for dinner in the summer, especially Irish oatmeal. People who need to lower their cholesterol may want to look into the benefits of oatmeal.

• Pumpkin seeds: I love to chew up the seeds and spit out the shells. Gross? Well, I don't do it in public! And it really is a healthy way for me to satisfy my taste buds when I want something salty. Popping pumpkin seeds is also a great way to gift your body with copper, iron, magnesium, manganese, phosphorus, and the prostate-protecting mineral zinc.

• Salmon: I make a blackened-salmon salad that's jamming. I can have salmon for breakfast, lunch, and dinner—anytime. It is my all-time favorite fish. Because salmon is rich in omega-3 essential fatty acids, many rate it a top heart-healthy food. Salmon's other offerings include vitamins B_6 and B_{12}.

• Soy: I love chocolate soy milk; I even have my husband drinking soy milk, and he loves it. And I love soybeans. My family has not quite acquired the taste for edamame—oh, well, more soy for me! In moderation, however, the rule of thumb for just about all foods. At one point, I thought my breasts were falling off, they hurt so bad. Off I went for a mammogram. Thankfully, no breast cancer. Still, I was told to ease up on my soy consumption because, for me, breast pain is a side effect of consuming too much.

• Spinach: Spinach is one of my choice veggies. I learned to incorporate it into almost any meal, including breakfast. I sauté fresh spinach (so it doesn't get soggy) with a bit of fresh minced garlic, a little chopped fresh green onion, and add a little Mrs. Dash seasoning. Then I scramble everything together with an egg sub-

stitute, maybe add a little salsa, and voilà! Your digestive, lymphatic, and urinary systems will thank you for
eating spinach.

• Tea: Green tea tops black tea, many people say.
When I feel I need a little help eliminating, I find that
drinking a cup a night for three nights running gets me
clean as a whistle.

• Tomatoes: I eat tomatoes like fruit—well, they *are*
fruit. They have seeds. They also have vitamin A, vitamin
C, calcium, and the antioxidant lycopene.

• Turkey: I make grilled turkey thighs that taste like
pork. Turkey thighs—oh, what a discovery! I can jerk
'em, smoke 'em, grill 'em, and bake 'em in a bag, a real
paper bag. You can take the most inexpensive parts of
a turkey, season them up, put them in a paper bag, and
have some good eats when done—and it's leaner than
other meats.

• Walnuts: I confess I am not a walnut fan, but many
people looking to lower their cholesterol have made
this nut their snack and started adding them to their
salads and other dishes.

• Yogurt: You can use yogurt instead of sour cream to
reduce calories in a recipe. Among other things, yogurt contributes to colon health.

Ultimately, we are responsible for what we do with our lives, and we have the power to take control of our lifestyles and fashion them as we want for better or worse. So I don't blame my parents or my environment for all the bad habits I cultivated early on in my life—and continued for way too long. But over the days, as I sipped my two ounces of water, or two ounces of juice, or two ounces of protein shake, and as I reflected on all my years of battling diabetes, of holding up on weak knees, of getting winded so easily, of fearing an early grave, of being so miserable physically so many of my days—as I reckoned with this drastic journey of gastric bypass, I could not help but think and know, *This did not have to be! If only . . . If only I knew then what I know now.* Then again, as Søren Kierkegaard said, "Life can only be understood backwards, but must be lived forward." And that's what I was determined to do.

In mid-August 2003 I entered phase III, with full liquids added to my meal plan for breakfast, lunch, and dinner. My options consisted of pure fruit and vegetable juices; nonfat custard; sugar-free, fat-free gelatin or pudding; low-fat or nonfat plain yogurt; cream of wheat or cream of rice cereal; and soups strained thin or creamed.

Because I am dairy intolerant, I had to forget about some of the items on the plan. Before the surgery, I occasionally allowed myself some dairy, aided by an enzyme to help me digest it—lactase, in supplement form or in milk products like Lactaid. But after the surgery, with my digestive system so compromised, I cut out all dairy until I healed completely. (Cheese! I missed cheese!)

Now that I had entered phase III, it was time to get back in the mix. My very first public appearance, thanks to an invite from one of my girlfriends, was in late August, ironically to see an August. It was an afternoon affair honoring the playwright August Wilson. By then I had dropped about forty pounds. (I was losing ten pounds a week the first few weeks.) I was nervous. I did not know how people would relate to me after all the years of my being the fat, jolly Mother Love—the safe Mother Love. How would they feel about the changing Mother Love? What would they ask me? How would I respond? Especially in the entertainment business, when people see someone who has lost a lot of weight, the first thing they think is crack cocaine or AIDS. And indeed, months after my surgery, when I was in a restaurant in Vegas, a man shouted out, "Damn, Mother Love, you so little! You got AIDS?"

No one at the August Wilson affair was so rude. When someone remarked or inquired about my weight loss, I kept it simple. In response to the question "What's with the little cup?" I replied that I was on a superstrict regimen to combat my diabetes. When someone said, "Oh, you look great!" I said, "More important, I feel so much better, and I am so much healthier." I felt that my gastric bypass surgery was nobody's business! That was too personal to talk about with mere acquaintances and total strangers! I had likened it to asking a woman if she was on her period or a guy if he had jock itch.

Thankfully, I have girlfriends I could talk with about the details of my life change—including the gross side of bypass. When you don't eat a lot, you don't poop a lot. I really thought I was going to die when I could not have a proper bowel movement. Early on, it was hell. It was like trying to crap a brick. It was long, hard, and painful. I was crying and screaming and scaring everybody in the house. I was in agony. I did not have enough fluid in my intestinal tract to properly lubricate movement. I could not drink enough water to get that movement. You know how bad you feel and how bad your breath can smell when you cannot take a crap! I finally had to call the doctor. He said I could take a little bit of Milk of Magnesia. I am telling you: there is a very real ugly part of obesity surgery. I had to take ursodiol (the generic form of Actigall) for six months after the surgery to guard against gallstones, a possible consequence of rapid weight loss. A drastic drop in pounds changes your bile mixture, and, as my MD told me, there is a 30 percent chance of developing gallstones because of this alteration in bile mixture. The good news: if medication is introduced within the first few months, your chance of developing gallstones drops to 3 percent. I never developed gallstones.

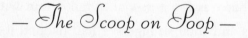

— *The Scoop on Poop* —

Ideally, we should have a bowel movement two to three times a day. Movements should occur shortly

after we have eaten a meal. There should be no strain-
ing. When your stool floats, you have been doing well.
Your stool should not be runny like diarrhea or in
clumps and lumps but loose and floating. It should
smell like what you have ingested.

I was actually living this new life away from home. In late
August 2003, I went to Atlanta to finish work on a few
scenes for the romantic comedy *Fair Game* as well as to do
some promo work on the film at an outdoor festival. The
film starred some of Hollywood's beautiful people: Gina
Torres (my baby boo and Laurence Fishburne's wife), Kellita
Smith (*The Bernie Mac Show*), Marc Christopher Lawrence
(*Christmas with the Kranks*), and fine Michael Jace (*The
Shield*). I played the love psychic and apartment owner who
hates the male romantic lead played by my friend Michael
Whaley, who also directed the film. Because I had lost forty
pounds, when it came to finishing those few scenes, it was a
continuity nightmare, but Michael found a way to make it all
work.

In early September I went into phase IV of my must,
must, *must* healing plan. At last! For breakfast, lunch, and dinner some food I could sink my teeth into!—kinda sorta. It was
baby food. For breakfast: one ounce (two tablespoons) of a
high-protein food, a half ounce of fruit, and a half ounce of
starch. For lunch and dinner: one ounce of a high-protein
food; a half ounce of veggie; and a half ounce of starch or fruit.

The high-protein food list included pureed fish and meats; scrambled or pureed eggs; and several things I could not have due to lactose intolerance: cottage cheese, cream soups, yogurt, milk. For the fruit, it was take your pick—so long as it was pureed. Veggies? Whatever I wanted, just so long as it was pureed. And not gas forming. So I could say yes to carrots, green beans, squash, and such, but unless I wanted to be in a great deal of discomfort, I had to say no to the likes of broccoli, cauliflower, lettuce, spinach, and cabbage. Until I healed, such gas-producing veggies would put too much strain on my little pouch.

For starches, it was more of the same from phase III plus the options of rice, pasta, and baby-soft mashed potatoes or yams. I was glad that I could eat some food with a bit more heft, but that baby food was icky; so flavorless. I understood why babies make that face when they see baby food coming toward them. I started pureeing my own food.

I shouted glory hallelujah when later in the month I was able to move up to solid food for my three main meals a day—but still only two ounces per meal for the first two weeks. In time I was able to increase my intake. Soon I was able to eat pretty much whatever I prepared for my family, only never in the quantity that they could handle. Their meals I served on dinner plates; my half-a-sandwich-worth (about six ounces), on a salad plate.

Once I was back on solid food, I chose not to eat bread for a while. With my intake capacity so severely reduced, I knew bread, especially bread with yeast, would get me full quicker than veggies or protein. I needed the nutritional benefits of the latter more than I needed the pleasure of bread. Plus, chewing bread thoroughly is more of a challenge. When I began to allow myself bread, I limited it to flatbreads: pita and other yeastless types. I sometimes even make my own bread to avoid additives and preservatives that often come in store-bought bread. I learned the hard way that I cannot partake of my corn-bread stuffing. During one postsurgery Thanksgiving dinner, two small forkfuls of stuffing left me unable to eat the rest of the ounces of food on my little plate. I felt as if I had a brick in my stomach.

— *Bookin'* —

I am a cookbook fanatic. I read cookbooks to see what I like, what I can modify to fit my meal plans, as well as for ideas for new creations. Below are a few of the books I keep at the ready by my stove. Many people who enjoy meals at my house cannot believe that they are eating low fat and virtually sugar free.

• *1000 Low Fat, Salt, Sugar & Cholesterol Recipes to Tempt Your Tastebuds.* As of this writing, I have been through about 150 of the recipes.

• *The New Soul Food Cookbook for People with Diabetes* by Fabiola Demps Gaines and Roniece Weaver. I always wanted to write a book like this. I may not have to. Fabiola and Roniece's recipes are easy to prepare and do not require you to go to some specialty store for ingredients. The authors provide the American Diabetes Association's food-exchange guidelines for each dish. I'm also partial to the book because Fabiola looks like one of my aunties.

• *The Diabetic's Healthy Exchanges Cookbook* by JoAnna M. Lund. "Real food for people living in the real world with diabetes" is the book's tagline. Real true!

• *The Healing Foods: The Ultimate Authority on the Creative Power of Nutrition* by Patricia Hausman and Judith Benn Hurley. I picked up this book after I moved to L.A. and before I was diagnosed with diabetes. What drew me to the book was my desire to glean information to pass on to my family in Cleveland. They ignored the information. But no good thing ever goes to waste: the book really helped me. Through it, I became convinced that cures for many ailments can be found in plants and root things.

By late fall 2003, I was in full compliance with the post-surgery plan, including exercise. "Exercise during rapid weight loss is critical to redirect your body to use up fat stores rather than valuable proteins," explained the booklet Dr. Lourie had given me. "You will need to plan for a minimum of twenty minutes of aerobic exercise a day to ensure healthy weight loss." I started exercising about two weeks after my surgery, when my doctor said it was safe to do so. I chose morning swims. Early on, it was really more like a morning walk in the water: walking up, back, and across in the pool for twenty minutes. I added water weights as I got stronger. After about a month or so of this, I was able to add laps. In time, I was swimming every morning for about an hour, with rest stops.

There came a day when I found myself actually bounding up and down stairs with ease. When I was limited to a parking space far from a store entrance, I did not mind at all. It felt good to walk. It felt good to be in better health, in a better place. I was surprised I did not miss too much food. Oh, I missed a piece of cake here, a piece of cheese there—but I was working it! And, thankfully, I never had that Henry the Eighth dream again.

Yes, I was feeling so much better, but let me be clear: my life was not easier. It's not easy to follow such a superstrict eating regimen. It's not easy to eat out with other people. I have to scrutinize a menu so much longer than before, analyzing it for what I can eat with ease, asking questions of waiters—"Is this cooked in butter?" I have to keep myself from getting cranky or envious of tablemates who order things I cannot: like the time I was in a trendy New York City restaurant having lunch with my son and two colleagues. Each one of them decided on a Cuban sandwich, while I ordered small portions of a few things, sautéed mushrooms among them. The way they ate, I could tell their sandwiches were scrumpdelicious. Had I not given up pork so many moons before I had the surgery, my envy might have been quite acute.

And then there's the *time* factor: because just about everyone I know eats faster than I can afford to, it's not always easy for me to keep myself from speed eating. I have learned to say, "I will need a 'to go' box." What helps are memories of what happened when I slipped up. When I ate too fast and ended up with the shakes and sweating like a pig. When I ate and drank too closely together and ended up dumping.

When my eating so selectively and so slowly, in such small portions, raised eyebrows, my standard line became, "I have diabetes, and I must eat a certain way." It was still much simpler than saying, "I had gastric bypass, and I can only eat a small amount." It seemed to me that folks would take my having a debilitating disease a lot easier than my drastic action. And I repeat: obesity surgery is drastic! Had I found another way, I would not have had that surgery. Better is good, but I repeat: better is not easy. "You did well today," self would say to self at the end of a day. "More work tomorrow." I knew that tomorrow would be better, but not easy.

"Not easy" is a concept many people have trouble accepting, especially in America. Most Americans believe they are entitled to easy. But in many respects, easy is not better. Using spell-check is easier than proofing your writing the old-fashioned way—with your two eyes and your mind. But doesn't it make our mental muscle a bit flabby? Allowing children to hole up in their rooms watching TV or playing video games for hours on end is easy but not in the child's best interest. "At least he's not running the streets," you may say. True. He may even be improving his hand-eye coordination. But if he's playing violent games, he may also be desensitizing his soul. What's more, when it's time for the child to study for an algebra test or write an essay, he may not be able to focus on the task because things aren't exciting enough for him, not moving fast enough.

It's easy and getting easier to feed children and ourselves fast food and microwave meals than it is to shop for fresh food and prepare it with an eye on optimum nutrition. Taking a pill for what ails you is easier than changing your diet and trading time before the tube for time on the treadmill. Plunking down plastic is easier than saving up and paying cash. But all this easy is making our lives more difficult on some levels.

— Save the Children —

• In 1990 less than 4 percent of American children and teens were diagnosed with type 2 diabetes. A decade later, that number had more than quadrupled.

• The majority of young people diagnosed with type 2 diabetes are overweight or obese at the time of their diagnosis.

- Young people of color are more likely to contract type 2 diabetes than are Caucasian children.

- The Centers for Disease Control and Prevention has predicted that one out of every three Americans born in 2000 is at risk of being a type 2 diabetic by 2025.

Many a night, as I drifted off to sleep, faces of certain friends and relatives flashed on my mental screen. In my spirit, I screamed, "Do something now! Don't wait until your eyesight is compromised, you're peeing all day long, you're up changing the sheets in the middle of the night, cannot quench your thirst, or, worse, your kidneys are failing!"

After my surgery, I continued to urge certain family members to change their ways—quit smoking, quit drinking, quit eating so much killing food, and quit saying, "It's just a little sugar." A few family members and friends listened up, I'm happy to report. One began eating as I do. She lost thirty pounds in the first three months of her modified meal plans and portion control. Sadly, not everyone heeded my urging to change their ways.

It really broke my heart that my baby sister, Brenda, was unable to change her ways for her health's sake. Because she had not, in late November 2003—seven months after Paula's death, four months after I had gastric bypass—Brenda checked into the hospital to have her left leg amputated from the knee down. That's how bad the circulation in that leg had gotten.

I went to see my sister before her surgery. She was terrified. She cried uncontrollably in my arms. As I held and rocked her gently, my husband prettied up her hospital room with flowers and pictures of our grandson, whom she had yet to meet. My sister's doctor told me that her failure to stop smoking was why she lost her leg so soon.

Brenda quit smoking long enough to get her leg amputated, heal, and get home. And after her amputation, she was back with her packs. I was so furious with her. She had a daughter who needed her mother—and a whole lot of other family who wanted her to be around longer. But she, in her early forties, was looking like she had one foot in the grave. The one that had been on a banana peel was gone.

As with my older sister's death, my baby sister's amputation was another powerful, painful reminder of the consequences of not making the shift—and how grateful to GOD I was that I had been able to do it. Celebrate? Oh, yes! I had a birthday coming up.

– 9 –
A VERY HAPPY BIRTHDAY!

I was going to make it to fifty after all—and in better shape than I had been in for a very long time. I had finally gotten that weight off. I continued to swim in the mornings and added walks to my evenings. *I am going to live*, I constantly thought. "Focus on wellness, not illness," says Dr. James Gavin III in his book *Dr. Gavin's Health Guide for African Americans.* That's absolutely what I was doing—focusing on my wellness. And it was time to party!

My fiftieth birthday party had been on my mind, marinating, for a few years. I first caught the vision in early 2000. Later I started my fiftieth-birthday-party fund. I earmarked residual checks for it. I had started doing stand-up again to keep my chops honed. When I started to get paid for it again, I started doing it more for the sake of my birthday fund. I did not want to pinch off bill money. I did not want to put my party on plastic. I wanted this party to be free and clear. After folks ate up all the food, drank up all the liquor, danced, laughed, joked, talked, and made new connections—pay finance charges on the memories? I don't think so.

With my birthday being December 29, and 2004 kicking in a few days later, I decided to have my party on New Year's Eve. I had a fine time making the invitations. (I am dangerous with a glue gun!) And folks still have those invitations hanging on their bulletin boards. OK, maybe just my family in Cleveland.

When I mailed the invitations, I knew that few of those relatives would attend my party. Some simply did not fly. Others could not afford to make the trip. Some who had the money just were not going to spend it to see me. Several family members actually said they would happily come to my party, but only on my nickel. They wanted me to pay for their tickets, put them up, and feed them. Because the invitations looked as if they cost a fortune, they believed I could easily afford to send for them. I told them I made the invitations.

As for the other people on my guest list, folks were actually RSVP'ing! Most people I know *never* RSVP. They just show up, bring their friends, bring a container in which to take food home, and then don't want to go home. But this time, I guess they RSVP'd because they saw that my party was going to be a very classy affair; they knew they needed to act right!

I had booked a hotel ballroom, hired a swank jazz trio for the cocktail hour, and a funky band, plus a DJ. I had found the perfect caterer to do the food like I eat: low fat, sugar free, *and* yumptious. Oh, the drinks were going to flow, and I was going to glow—like a happy pregnant woman glows! Remember, this was a New Year's Eve party, so I had to pay premium prices. Did I flinch at the money I had to dole out in deposits? Oh, no! No problem! I got the chips. "I am ret ta go!"

I was bopping around like a schoolgirl getting ready for a first date. I was giddy for weeks, planning the menus, preparing the music list for the DJ, and designing the centerpieces. When it came to concocting a specialty drink, I called on three girlfriends with discerning palates to come over to my house to test my mixes. I mixed apple, peach, and other flavored martinis. I made the drink called Beautiful (Grand Marnier and Courvoisier Cognac). One teeny taste of that drink made my knees hot. (All hard liquor makes my knees hot; that's why I don't drink it.) I mixed up another drink: "Add gin, vodka, and tequila with some margarita mix, and let's see what that tastes like!" My friends thought it tasted pretty good. They also thought it would get people pretty drunk—and you know how folks are when booze is free. Plus, in my community, if you have a party, and somebody gets drunk at your house and

afterward gets behind the wheel of a car and into a car accident, you could be held responsible. I wanted folks to have a
good time, not catch a case. In the end, I chose apple martinis
with a slice of green apple as the specialty drink.

As guests pulled up to the hotel, they would be greeted by
a doorman and treated to valet parking. My interns, dressed in
red and black, would escort guests into the cocktail-hour
room. Everyone who had RSVP'd would be grandly an-
nounced at the entrance. It was going to be hilarious to see
everybody's reaction to a stately man calling out their names,
followed by a burst of applause.

The jazz trio would be jamming. The specialty drinks,
mixed to perfection. The hors d'oeuvres—Asian spring rolls,
chicken and shrimp wontons, and one of my favorite foods,
Buffalo wings—sumptuous. Guests would mingle, exchange
business cards (they would do it anyway, so I'd let them
know it was all right), and make new friends. At the dinner
hour, a very elegant man in full tuxedo would announce,
"Dinner is now being served."

Guests would be ushered into a room with an archway of
black, red, gold, and purple balloons. They'd see black tablecloths sprinkled with multicolored confetti and adorned
with centerpieces of red roses, gold carnations, and those little purple flowers that grow all over California.

I was going to make my entrance in a red, slinky spa-
ghetti-strapped little number with a pair of red-hot strappy
three-inch stiletto shoes. My toes would be well pedicured.
I'd even get a set of nails put on my toes, so they would be

toe-sucking ready! I was down to 170 pounds by then. I had gone from size 22 to size 12! I was going to have everybody screaming when the stately man introduced me: "Ladies and Gentlemen . . . the even more fabulous . . . Mother Love!"

I would glide ever so sexily down the staircase. When I entered the cocktail room, I'd hug and kiss everyone, then make my way to the mike to formally welcome my guests. You know I would have to say *something.* It's my party, and I'll talk if I want to, talk if I want to.

My guests were going to dine on blackened salmon, fresh assorted grilled vegetables (zucchini, yellow squash, carrots), a salad of mixed greens with low-fat dressing, and garlic red potatoes. For dessert: berry tarts and assorted sorbets. For a buzz: Corona beer (the beer I'd drink if I drank beer) and quite pricey red and white wines. Few if any guests would know that all the food was chosen and prepared in keeping with my diabetic meal plan. Well, all except for the booze. It was a party, after all, and most of the people I know drink.

Several video cameras would be strategically placed in my birthday party space to capture all the excitement from the time people entered the door until they left. And music would not be the only live entertainment. I had auditioned several stand-up comics before—*Duh?* I called up my nephew in Cleveland, who is following me into show business. He, aka, CeeTown, was ret ta go!

The closer the date, the giddier I got. Then, one day in mid-November the phone rang—my gid hit a skid. My son was in a car accident. Front end crushed, tire balled up, both air bags deployed. He had torn up his car! It was a miracle that he emerged uninjured, only badly shaken up.

You never really know what people are hiding until they get into trouble or die. Well, Jahmal was in a heap of trouble. When the cops came on the scene, they ran his plates and license. Uh-oh. Jahmal had unpaid tickets for driving without being buckled up, for driving without his license. So my son got a taste of the slammer. Kennedy was the one who went to get him out of jail. I didn't go because I know when it's man-to-man time. But I wish I could have been a fly on the dashboard during *that* ride home. I don't know what Kennedy said to Jahmal, but it must have been some powerful words given how truly contrite our son was when they got home.

The whole debacle ended up costing Jahmal more than fifteen thousand dollars. His smallest expense was the three hundred dollars for the pole he hit. (He didn't want to file an insurance claim. He felt it would be better to eat the costs than see his premium skyrocket.) Making matters worse, Jahmal was several thousand dollars in debt before the accident. For starters, he still had a note on the 2000 Taurus he had wrecked. He could have paid the car off a long time ago. He was just a young buck with a head like a brick, ignoring Kennedy and me all the while we were riding him: save money, save money! (That's another book: *Teaching Our Children Fiscal Responsibility, or, Stop Pimping the 'Rents.*)

I was furious with Jahmal—but I am his mother. How

could I have my swanky-swank birthday party in light of his situation? I went to my birthday fund and lent him the cash. As of this writing, my son has paid me back some of the money, six grand, and I am not letting him off the hook! I want the rest of my dough. The moral? When you embark on a journey to wellness, you have to be prepared for bumps along the way—especially obstacles and frustrations not of your making. You have to have a special mantra or prayer for such times, a booster that will help you to keep moving forward. It also helps to have a few true-true friends.

After I raided my birthday fund for my son, I called three of my aces in Cleveland on a three-way. When Lori, Derellya, and Bobette got on the line with me, I was crying like a baby about what I was gonna do. The invitations were mailed, deposits were in place. I was weeks away from my big dream of hosting the soiree of the year!

My friends let me vent and have my fit. When I shut up for a few seconds, I heard—

"Girl, you have all that pretty home. Have it there."

"You are turning fifty, and we are going to celebrate with you!"

Do you know the difference between a good friend and a great friend? "A good friend will help you move, a great friend will help you move the body." Lori, Derellya, and Bobette were willing to help me move the body. Or, as one of them put it, "Girl, we got you! We will come in early and help you."

Lori, Derellya, and Bobette had their thinking caps on.

They told me to whittle the guest list down to just my true friends, the ones who would not get bent out of shape over a change in plans, the ones who would be happy to celebrate with me at a bowling alley. They reminded me that they can all cook (no lie). All I had to do was show them how to make diabetic-friendly food. They reminded me that they have some skills when it comes to decorating, too. All I had to do was give them a nudge in the direction I wanted them to go and "We can put it together!" My friends had me so pumped. But then I thought, *Ain't it kinda tacky to uninvite people—to call up and say, "Guess what, I can't do the swanky-swank"*? My girlfriends asked what was more important: being tacky or having a big fat debt if I went ahead with the swanky-swank? *I can do tacky,* I thought.

It was still going to be a great party. Only now, one big house party! And I was blessed to get a refund on some of the deposits. The hotel manager was really cool with the refund because I had rented the big ballroom on several other occasions.

Next, I had to pare down the guest list and change the venue from the hotel to our home. I didn't realize how cluttered my life was with casual people, folk who just wanted to hang out with me and on to me but who had no real relationship with me other than, "I know Mother Love" BS. My guest list dropped from four hundred to one hundred. After I let the one hundred know about the change of venue, I got down to the fun part! I started re-visioning my re–birthday party.

I ordered a tent to cover my driveway and had my garage cleared out so I could transform it into a dance floor. I cut bait on the jazz trio but kept the funky band. Had I canceled them, I would have still had to pay them their full fee because it was a New Year's Eve booking and it was too late for them to get booked somewhere else on such short notice. I did not mind. I would hire them today.

There were round tables and red tablecloths to rent along with black lacquered chairs, which had to be padded. Like me, most of my friends are over forty. There is nothing like going to an event where the chairs are so hard that your butt goes numb on one side after sitting for a while. Besides, with no more cushy tushy, my coccyx was hurting all the time. Old injury from Mr. Teacher.

OK, so I would not use a florist. Instead, I'd go to the L.A. flower mart at o'dark-thirty the morning of the party to buy flowers. My assistant, Alan, had graciously offered to create arrangements for placement here and there around the house. One arrangement was a masterpiece of swirling branches, my beloved tiger lilies, and other posies for the big table in our foyer. He is so very creative! Instead of having floral centerpieces, I decided to make something. I transformed eight-inch lady mannequins into little queens.

Lori, Derellya, and Bobette were true to their word. They arrived in L.A. several days before my party. Plus, Derellya brought her fella. Plus, my nephew CeeTown came in early, too! Everybody was ready to get to work, as were my husband and son. Four fellas for hauling, lifting, and

moving. We ladies for the catering and decorating commit-
tee. Still, at turns, I was a basket case: "Can we get it done?"
Everyone's attitude was essentially, "Yes, woman—if you
stop tripping!"

We started food prep the night before, on New Year's
Eve eve. We prepared relish trays and vegetable trays; made a
raspberry yogurt dip; mixed up pasta salad; rolled assorted
turkey cold cuts; and whipped up a low-fat ranch dressing
for dipping the Buffalo wings we were cooking up—no, not
deep fried, but grilled, then dipped into the hot sauce (and
no one was the wiser). We also hooked up the mac and
cheese and some finger-licking jerk turkey. All the while, we
laughed, joked, reminisced—had a blast.

The centerpiece of the menu was one of my recent creations: hot and sassy cabbage and shrimp with black beans
and a Zatarain's rice mix, and corn muffins—from scratch!
When I first told people about my cabbage and shrimp dish,
most of them said, "*Yew*, shrimp and cabbage?" But after
they'd tried it, I'd get calls about it. "Hey, Mother Love, when
are ya making that shrimp and cabbage again?"

As there were four women in the kitchen, we got finished early and we figured we deserved a night out on the
town. We gals got dolled up; the fellas fixed up fly. We ended
up at a club where one of my favorite bands, Funjala, was
playing. The bandleader, Victor Orlando, made us his guests.

CeeTown was all over the dance floor as the rest of us
headed upstairs to the club's VIP section. As I looked at all
the action on the floor, the new and improved me kicked in.

I may be too old to go clubbing every night but I am by no means ready for the porch. I grabbed my husband, and we headed downstairs to hit the dance floor. I was dropping it like it's hot. I couldn't pick it up, but I could drop it.

The next day was decoration time—I was a neurotic mess. What if it rains? What if it's too cold for people to be outside even though we had the large patio heaters? I was going crazy with the what-ifs. I was crying and snapping at everybody. By then, that everybody included California girl-friends Kathy, Cynthia, An, and my assistant. At one point everybody was like, Enough! They told my husband to take me somewhere, anywhere, because I was getting on their nerves. What did my husband do? What every husband should do when his wife is tripping: take her shopping! I can have a good time shopping for tires.

When we returned home, I was cool, calm, and collected. When I walked into my house, I was flabbergasted. My dear, darling friends had worked some beautiful magic. You would have thought I had paid a high-end professional party deco-rator to do the job. When I stepped into the kitchen, I saw that they had gone through all the cabinets and closets and found bowls, serving trays, and pretty glasses—things I had forgotten we owned.

I lost it when I went into my driveway-turned-dining-room and saw that they'd placed photographs of family members on the tables, including those of my parents and others who could be there only in spirit. At that point, I knew that everything was going to be OK. If it rained, if the temperature dropped—no matter what: I was going to have a very happy birthday party. Not even the DJ drama could steal my joy.

The DJ was a gift from my California friend Cynthia. At a moment when my head wasn't on straight, I had canceled the DJ I had booked for my swanky-swank, even though I had paid him in full. Oh, well. Anyway, the DJ Cynthia booked didn't connect with her to get my address and directions until the morning of the party. After she gave him the details, she added, "Let me give you Mother Love's cell phone number in case you get lost or something."

"Mother Love? Mother Love-Mother Love? The real Mother Love?" My friend said he sounded very excited.

"Yes, the real Mother Love," she replied. "It's her big birthday bash."

"I have to call you back," Mr. DJ said. As it turned out, he was more than excited. He was greedy. When Mr. DJ called Cynthia back, he tripled his price! "Well, it's for a celebrity. Plus, it's New Year's Eve—too late to book somebody else, so you either pay my fee, or you will not have a DJ." Cynthia told him she would have to get back to him. She then phoned me.

Cynthia wanted to wring his neck and tell him, hell no! but she told me that if I really wanted a DJ, she was willing to give in to his demand. I was like, hell no! I told her we could simply turn the TV on to a music station, put some fabric over it, and call the DJ a D.A.Y. That ended up working very well.

People partied like you are supposed to at a house party,

getting hot and sweaty, getting loud from the laughter, staying into the wee hours like my house was their home. My hot and sassy cabbage and shrimp dish was a big hit. When it ran out, my girlfriend An put on an apron and helped me make another and bigger batch.

Just as I had planned for my swanky-swanky, I was the woman in red. I modified the outfit because the night was too chilly for a barely there dress. I wore a black skirt with a handkerchief bottom and an adorable off-the-shoulder red sweater with black lace trim that made me look like I'd had a boob job. The "girls" were perky.

I was one very grateful woman that night. I had survived the surgery; I had stayed with the post-op plan. I was moving around easier. I was no longer scared. And I was celebrating with a great crowd of family and friends. What a way to ring in the new year. We'd had a prayer before the party. We all stood around the kitchen holding hands. We gave thanks and shared our hopes for the coming year. To have all those people in my life who love me in spite of myself, big or small, is a beautiful feeling.

I was grateful for the presents, too! Everyone who knows me knows I love presents. They cannot come to a party I throw without a present. It does not have to be elaborate. I love and cherish handmade presents the most. For my birthday, I think I got about three vibrating foot massagers. I go to the nail salon about every two weeks. What was I going to do with all of them? Regift! (That's on the low, OK?)

My girlfriend Golden Girl, a boxer, gave me an enchanting ceramic butterfly box. I also received a beautiful edition of the Holy Bible, featuring great women of the Bible; a book about one of my heroes, Muhammad Ali; and a book of romantic poetry by Nelson Brown, an L.A.-based writer whose previous book, *Whispers in My Ear*, was the basis of his spoken-word CD, *Naturally You*, on which I guest starred.

Knowing how much I love caricatures, Cynthia had booked one of L.A.'s premier artists to make caricatures for my guests. She also hired two masseuses to give complimentary shoulder and neck massages. The caricaturist set up in our formal living room; the masseuses, in our piano room. As we don't have a piano, I call it my "Mother Love to the Motherland" room. It contains artwork and other mementos from our trip to Dakar, Senegal.

People who did not attend my party, including some who had been canceled, sent gifts. There were cards with gift certificates to spas and trendy new restaurants. And I will never forget the gift my beloved cousin Tootie sent: fifty dollars. I was really shocked because she is on a fixed income. When I called to thank her and to tell her that I was going to return her money, she would not hear of it. "We are family!" she said. "Go buy yourself a hat or something."

For years, when the holidays roll around, Kennedy and I have maintained the tradition of having folks who visit during the season sign and date our dining room tablecloth with glitter glue or puffy paint. People can write anything they want on the tablecloth, so long as it's not obscene. At my party in 2003, the cloth filled up quickly with birthday salutations and well wishes for the New Year.

One of the tablecloths in the tent had a very different ending. Somebody—and they have not been ratted out yet—accidentally set it on fire, so it had a huge burn on it. Instead of throwing it away, I let it be my new dining room tablecloth for the New Year. On it I wrote, "My 50th was so hot it was on fire!"

– 10 –

HOT MAMA LOVE?

So what you gonna do with your wife now?" That's what I heard a guy ask my husband as my party was winding down.

I wanted to tell him, "Hopefully the same thing he was doing with me before—only more, because I no longer get so winded."

What did that man think? That I would be on the prowl for a boy toy?

Some people had long wondered what the deal was with my husband and me. What does he see in her? They figured I had to be doing something to his food and water. I was too fat, too loud, too aggressive, cussed too much, talked too much mess. He, on the other hand, is the laid-back, quiet type. "Ain't gonna last," people had said. We've been getting that since 1972. When folks saw that our relationship endured for thirteen years before we married, then lasted another twentysomething years, some figured with all his quiet, something had to be wrong with him. Translation: a defective man was all fat-and-happy me could get. Now that I was no longer fat and so much happier, people figured it would only be a matter of time before I traded up. My husband would have to watch me like a hawk, they believed.

Our big problem was trying not to get pregnant. I was in perimenopause, and Dr. Lourie had said that I could have a fertility surge. He recommended that I take birth control pills for a while unless Kennedy and I wanted an Oops baby.

The more weight I lost, the weirder people got. Nonsense came my way from strangers, too. Offers poured in from companies hoping to make some bucks off the slimmed-down me. "We want you to be our spokesperson!"

There was a workout video. All I had to say was that the program was the secret of my weight-loss success, and they would pay me a half million dollars for starters. I received similar offers for a diet pill and a weight-loss beverage.

But that's not what I did!

One company with a line of foods to be sold through infomercials offered to pay off my house, all my bills, pay me a fat fee, and give me a royalty on every unit of food that sold.

All I had to do was be the pitchperson: tell the world that I knew from experience that their products were the real deal, a surefire thing for anyone looking to shed mucho weight. Translation: conspire with us to pull a fast one on the public. Work with us to put a lie on TV, and we will pay you well.

And I will end up in hell!

"You could make untold millions," they said.

But I'd be making untold millions on a lie. Don't get me wrong; I can be as unscrupulous as anyone else. But I do have two scruples and a couple or three morals that I will not cross the line on. Had I been willing to go along with one of the propositions, it would have been risky, on top of immoral. Remember: I was on the other side of fifty. I did not need the pressure of worrying about forgetting what was lie, what was truth. I could see it now:

"So you tried that so-and-so pill?"

"Hell, no." (Oops!)

"So that line of food was the thing that worked for you?"

"Never tasted it." (Oops!)

I've always been the what-comes-up-comes-out type, but when you are over fifty, the truth will come flying out your mouth before you know you've even formed the words. Especially when you are feeling good and feeling free within yourself.

The offers from companies was irritating and for a minute tempting, but not really problematic. I can't say the same for the stuff I got from some "friends."

"Oh, she thinks she's cute."

My thought: *No, not cute—too seasoned for cute. Even more fabulous!*

"Oh, she thinks she's better than us."

My thought: *No, not better—smarter, more driven.*

When I got down to about 165 pounds, my sisters Brenda and Marcia told me point-blank that they could not deal with me being so much smaller. Laura, from my support group, had been so right. I was very glad for the heads-up on people relating differently to me. Still, it hurt to discover that more than a few "friends" could not cope with my self-improvement crusade. One girlfriend—we had been friends since we were eleven years old—stopped speaking to me. She wanted absolutely nothing to do with me.

"I don't want you talking to her," Ex-friend told her daughter, with whom I was also close.

"But, Mommy, it's your issue. You're mad at her—I'm not." The young teen could not grasp the reason her mother was angry with me.

The mother had been talking about me like a dog. She told her daughter that I was trying to raise her, to steal her away from her family. Her head was really strange. She thought that I was going to leave my husband, or he would leave me, and when that happened, she was going to be all over him. Kennedy and I just laughed. I told her that if she thought she could pull him, "Take your best shot!" He told her that he was not interested in her or her type of woman because she was trifling and goalless. I had completely outgrown her, as she has refused to grow or grow up. Her loss.

"I don't see what you're saying about her, and I don't think it's fair," the woman's daughter told her. No matter how daughter tried to reason with mother, mother stuck to her script: I was persona non grata. Then she tried to put her daughter on a guilt trip. "If you got any loyalty to me, then you won't talk to her." Clearly, if I can tell you about their tug-of-war, the daughter and I did not remain incommunicado.

Another friend went by the wayside after she blew up at me for talking about how wonderful it was to feel that I had some control over my life.

"You saying I don't have control of my life?" she snapped.

I had said no such thing. And I was not going to take her BS. "If you feel bad about you because I'm taking control of my life, that's really on you," I told her straight out.

There are people who were in my mix for years who are no longer so. I was not going to put up with them giving me attitude and grief because I was no longer fat and unhealthy with them, like them. There were also people with whom I really wanted to remain friends but could not do so because all they did was bring me down. They applauded my success at improving my health but constantly followed that up with a clatter of complaint. Whine. Whine. Whine. One friend said that she didn't think she could muster the strength and determination to correct her lousy habits. Whine. Whine. Whine. Another friend said she wanted my advice, but really only wanted to cry, and moan, and whine, whine, whine about what she wished she could do. One of the last things I told her was, "Look, as Henry Ford said, 'You can't build a reputation on what you are going to do.'"

To stay on point, my attitude had to be that if a smaller, healthier Mother Love took some folks out of their comfort zone—oh, well. "Y'all can pack a lunch, kiss the side crack of my narrow ass, and walk out backward," I wanted to say to many a "friend." In my head, I shouted it from the rooftop. Contrary to popular belief, I can self-edit and control my mouth.

Some people think I have even gotten sharper, more brutally honest. I agree. But I don't think it's all about the weight loss and better health. I think it's about turning fifty—a very liberating event. You are simply not as needy. Even if you are in the best of health, you realize that you will probably not live as long as you have already lived. That reality makes you increasingly intolerant of nonsense. Those adages about making the most of your time—every day, every hour, every minute—that stuff hits home.

"Your body has changed, but your essence, your spirit, has not changed at all." Those words came from a true friend. She was someone who really knew me and was not at all threatened by my success at increasing my chances of living longer—to see my grandson become a teenager, become a man; to feel myself walk up stairs with ease, to swim, to enjoy the quality of my life and others. With all the living I wanted to do, I could not afford to be cavalier about who I had in my inner circle.

There was a time when I let people choose to have me in

their lives because I never wanted to pursue a friendship and be rejected. When I was about eight and relatively new to Carver Park Estates, there was a girl about my age with whom I wanted to be friends so bad. She seemed like a nice girl, and she had a lot of brothers and sisters, but they didn't act as if they wanted to play with her. That inspired me to want to be her friend, make her my number-one playmate. She did not want to be my friend. In fact, she used to beat me up damn near every time I tried to talk to her. No matter what I did, she did not want to be my friend. I was crushed—and fool me was still wanting to be that girl's friend when I went off to college. How sick is that? The same thing happened to me a couple of times in college: when I pursued a friendship—rejection. Of course, by then I was too big for them to beat me up. To avoid being rejected, I started letting people choose me. I was a great cultivator but afraid to initiate. My husband is the only person I ever pursued as an adult.

As I continued to be a great cultivator, I also became an initiator after I turned fifty. I started choosing who I wanted in my life, and I became much more selective. If I pursue a friendship with someone who rejects me—crushed? I doubt it. Not after all that I have been through, not after getting a second chance, a profoundly new lease on life—and we are all just leasing this life. We own nothing. So, be my friend, don't be my friend. Be happy I have changed, hate me for changing. Whatever. I will just keep moving on, moving up, going higher. I am a woman very much unafraid of what people think. Unafraid of who does not like me. Unafraid of speaking my mind even more than before, something I did not think possible.

Only in one arena am I still afraid: my fear of the Lord—but "fear" in the Old Testament sense. In awe of. For I am a witness to the power of prayer, obedience, and supplication. Yes, I did the research. Yes, I did the counseling. Yes, I followed through on the post-op plan. But I could not have done any of that without the Almighty's wind beneath my wings. That is why I insist on uppercasing the whole of the name: GOD.

When it came to people, I trusted that GOD would keep and send the right people into my life, the people I need to continue my journey. I remember finally catching up with one friend after I had dropped a mega amount of weight. "Oh, I've just been waiting to get this hug from you," she said. She was genuinely, sincerely, could-pass-a-polygraph-test happy for the Even More Fabulous Mother Love. She said I had always been an inspiration, but even more so now. To her I was still the same Mother Love I had always been. No, that's not quite true. I was different: I was half the mother, twice the love.

"Oh, now I can hit on you," said a guy I'd known for years. He was cocksure he had something I could be wanting. "Looks like we can't call you Mother Love anymore," he whispered. "We got to call you Mother Sexy—Hot Mama Love."

"Fool, get out my face."

– 11 –

I SAVED MORE THAN MY LIFE— I SAVE MONEY!

I never realized how much it costs to be a big girl until I started slimming down. I am not talking about medical expenses that accrued as a result of my lugging around more weight than my body could bear. I'm talking about all the money spent on everyday maintenance—from soap, deodorant, and makeup to toilet paper. Yes, toilet paper lasts longer than ever.

Before: I had it down to a fine science. I could go from bed to bathed and dressed in about twenty minutes. That's because I had my clothes ironed or steamed and laid out the night before. I sometimes deviated from the outfit I had selected, but that was rare.

After: I decide what I will look like for the day the morning of. With so much less territory to cover, it takes me even less time to shower, shampoo, and shine.

Before: It could have been five hundred degrees outside, and there I was in panty hose. I had to wear them to combat thunder-thigh friction. For big girls: if your thighs are still applauding, and you have to wear panty hose in the summer, turn them inside out, so they don't make that swishy sound—in any season.

After: I wear panty hose only when I want to. I buy fewer pairs, and when I do, I'm not paying that higher plus-size price. I can get them from a dollar store. I don't, but I could! Typically, when a large woman wants to dress well, she has to spend more money on her wardrobe than a small woman does. Plus-size clothes cost more. Skinny people can wear just about anything and look okay, and even look chic in inexpensive things. I don't think every woman can wear everything and look good in it. Not even skinny people. Leggings, spandex—need I say more?

Before: I was limited to shopping at the likes of Lane Bryant, Ashley Stewart, Salon Z at Saks Fifth Avenue, and one of my favorite stores, Burlington Coat Factory ("We're More Than Great Coats"). When someone said, "You look great; where did you get that outfit?" and I replied, "Burlington," they rolled their eyes and thought I was kidding. Good. More for me.

After: I can shop anywhere I want! And I still love Burlington.

After I lost about eighty pounds, my husband made me lighten my closets of my pretty plus-size clothes and shoes. I commandeered a large room at our neighborhood community center and transformed it into a bona fide boutique. We had racks upon racks of dresses, gowns, blouses, coats, suits and slacks, and tables laid out with slips and nearly new lotta-body—and expensive—brassieres. As my boobies were the only two suckers I trust, I had hoisted the girls in style. I also had my husband and son weed out their wardrobes, along with toys and clothes our grandson had outgrown. *Ka-ching!*

I also gave away piles of clothes. That was something I had been doing for years. For a while, I represented a plus-size clothing line, and they gave me thirty to forty dresses a month. My clothes had a three-wear shelf life. I could wear it on camera, to church, to a meeting or a meal, then it had to go. The three-wear rule was my husband's doing. Being the clotheshorse and shoe horse that I am, I could have kept everything. He tripped out one time because I was on TV twice in one day in the same Versace-looking jacket. Not the same outfit, just the same jacket. I didn't know a taped show and a live show would air on the same day. That's when my husband instituted the three-wear rule. And what a bonanza it was for my womenkin. They would literally fight over the boxes and boxes of clothes I shipped back to Cleveland. Several cousins used to comb magazines and other media outlets to see what I was wearing, and then they were off to see who could get to me first to ask for the outfits. My sister Marcia would call me and say, "I have first dibs on all your clothes and jewelry!"

As I slimmed down, family had a lot more clothes to fight over. Marcia put dibs on the mink coat my husband had given me for my forty-fifth birthday. She would call me up all nice and such, and wiggle her way around to the coat. She said I had better not give it to anyone else. My husband wanted to save it for the Mother Love Museum. I wanted to sell it on the internet. As time moved on, and my beautiful, very large coat remained in storage, not being worn, I reminded my husband that I really wanted to wear the coat when we traveled to cold-weather places; how it was a shame I wasn't wearing it—so let's just sell it! That was a complete no-go on the selling of Mother's Mink. After I got it out of storage for a New York trip during a very cold snap, Kennedy saw how difficult it was for me to maneuver with such a large garment. "Fine, get your coat cut down," he finally said. I went to the furrier the day I was to return to L.A., got measured, had my coat reconstructed—and I am too, too fabulous in that coat!

I also gave clothes to friends and to friends of friends. One friend of a friend was a single mother of three who had recently moved to L.A. She was unemployed, but she was no slacker. She was on the hunt for a corporate position but did not have appropriate clothes for interviews. I know how hard it is to find nice plus-size things. For someone with limited funds it is darn near impossible. So when my friend told me about the woman, "Sure, bring her over," I said. When the woman met me, she did not know I was Mother Love at first. She just couldn't believe her eyes. After she got over it, we got down to business, and she ended up with about ten outfits she could really use and absolutely adored. She was in tears. Before she left, she said the sweetest thing: "I want to be a strong black woman like you, Mother Love." And she's Latina! Told you it was really sweet.

I hadn't started selling and giving away loads of big-girl clothes right out the gate. At first I tried to work with my wardrobe. As I lost weight, I had my designer pieces and suits altered. I did not want to or could not let them go! There came a point where I had no choice. I had one gorgeous designer skirt I had paid a grip for—on sale at that. I loved that skirt! I felt Hollywood sexy in it. It was black with embroidered teal, yellow, and red flowers, and a to-die-for split in the back. Black bugle beads adorned the hem, just as they did the edges of the sexy teal sweater with which I paired it. You could not tell me anything when I stepped out in that big number. I was fabulous! The skirt had started out as a size 22. The first time I took it to my tailor, he downsized it to size 16; about six weeks later, to size 12. When I downsized to size 10, "There's no more taking up!" he said. "It will start to look really crazy. You stop shrinking!"

By then, my husband had turned into a shopping freak. We'd be on our way to a meeting or an outing and—

"Look at that dress in the window!" *Screech!* He'd stop, pull over, or back up. "I like that dress—go get that dress!" And I would. Then we'd pass another store. *Screech!* "Ooh, look at that suit! Go in that store!" It could be a teenybopper store with stuff I would not wear if I had a whole makeover from those extreme people.

Finally, I had to tell my husband, "Look, I know I have lost a lot of weight and can wear pretty much what I want, but I am not trying to look twenty-five, thirty-five, or even forty. I want to look like the superbad, fine, fit, and fabulous fifty-year-old queen I am!" He has since calmed down. I had to stop him with the hoochie look. I am a grown woman.

After I dropped several sizes, friends and relatives to whom I once shipped boxes and boxes of clothing started whining, "What are we gonna do for clothes now?" They had no intention of losing weight and so would not be able to wear my little three-wear clothes. I had not realized that so many were depending on the things I sent them. Some of them even shared with me that they rarely bought clothes because they knew about the three-wear shelf life on my work clothes. One of them told me that all she bought was undergarments.

Although I need a lot of clothes for my work, I tried not to go hog wild with the shopping. For the most part, I stuck with my MO: buying timeless pieces and sprinkling in a few trendy items as each new season rolls around. I admit there was one area where I went a little crazy: belts! A big-belted Mother Love looked more like a lassoed Mother Love. Plus, when I sat down, the fat pouch would reveal itself, and half my belly would sit in my lap.

After: When I got a waistline again, I bought chain belts, leather belts, multicolored belts, belts of every color, and one with XOXOs on it.

Before: I had only a few pairs of jeans at any given time because it was so hard to find a pair that fit well. I had a butt so large you could serve dinner for eight on it. Besides, I like dresses and suits.

After: I have lots and lots of jeans. I can wear designer jeans because I've lost my butt. Though I still prefer dresses and suits, I do enjoy being able to wear more jeans and slacks.

Before: I had given up wearing high heels for anything longer than a photo op because my back, knees, and hips ached constantly. When my doctor had told me, "Your cute-shoes-wearing days are over," I wanted him dead right then. You cannot tell a shoe fanatic, "No high heels!"

After: I step often in three- and four-inch makes-you-wanna-holler CFMPs. OK, they still make my knees wanna holler, and wearing high heels remains an addiction I've yet to kick. I started so young. At age fourteen, I had my first little job. I spent almost all of my first few paychecks on a pair of $125 high heels I had seen in a fashion magazine. (Remember: this was in the 1960s.)

Before: One of my standard fat jokes was that when I died, I was coming back as a neck. I had a head and then shoulders but no neck. I often daydreamed about how it would feel to wear a choker again.

After: I have a neck! I can wear just about any kind of collar, from turtleneck and bateau to Dracula-like. And lo and behold, chokers came back. I have several chokers now. One of my new girlfriends, Linda G., gave me a custom-made black leather choker with Mother ♥ in the center. She always brings me the nicest, most thoughtful gifts. Thank you, girl.

And, oh, the wighats! And you know my hair is an accessory. I always wear hair to match my outfit or my mood. Now that I have a neck, I wear wighats I never dared put on my head. I even treated myself to a blond, braided, short wighat and a dark-brown spiky one.

Having a neck means I am no longer limited to studs and little hoops in my ears. I can wear ghetto-fabulous hoops; I can wear chandeliers; I can wear two earrings in one ear.

Before: If you looked at me straight on, you could not see both my ears.

After: You can see my whole head and both ears at once without moving around me.

Before: On long flights, the traveling mercies for which I prayed included, "Lord, please don't let me have to pee!" What knucklehead came up with that idea of going in such a tiny space? And my flying first class was only one part queen. Coach seats are made for little butts!

Before: I did not remember that beneath all the fat I had beautiful shoulders.

Before: I could not cross my legs under tables.

After: Now I can do that and more—wrap one foot

around the ankle of the other, like I did as a kid. And when I want to, I can do the hula hoop again!

— *My Pounding Down* —

July 2003	257 pounds
August 2003	207 pounds
December 2003	170 pounds
March 2004	146 pounds—my wellness weight!

Not all the "after" is a picnic. When I gave up the fat, I gave up cleavage. I went from sister full bosom to a sister with Raisinettes. I could carry everything up there before. I used to carry my money in my bosom: my "Twin City Bank." I could even carry loose change. Now I would have to tape money to my bra. I really miss my large breasts and my bodacious cleavage. Getting comfortable in the skin I was in took some time.

When you lose weight, all that skin that once bulged with fat does not disappear. There's much sagging and overlapping. Much tightening and toning to do! At first I was very self-conscious about my flabby upper arms. I really have some flags flying from the back of my once meaty arms. But I got over that. Now I'll go sleeveless in a heartbeat. And I picked up a tic: When riding in a car or sitting around running my mouth with friends, I got into the habit of playing with the flaps on my arms, pulling on them like some people twirl their hair. "Quit flipping your flags, Ma!" my son sometimes chided me, reminding me that pulling, flipping, and flicking the flap would make my arms flap and swag even more.

Though clothes shopping has become easier, in a sense it is not better—precisely because it is so easy. I often miss the challenge inherent in shopping for excellent and flattering big-girl clothes. I also miss not being able to carry big prints as well. I really look wild if the print is too busy.

People often tell me I look ten, twenty years younger. I think they are not looking at me with their good eye. I do not see what they see. Before, with a big, fat face, I had more of a baby face. I looked like thirty-five when I was forty-five. As I watched myself shrink, I said good-bye to short, fat fingers and hello to longer-looking fingers but older-looking hands. They had wrinkles, like other parts of me once kept wrinkle free because of the fat. I am just keeping it real: under my clothes, I look like a Shar-Pei. Short anything will not be on this body. My butt is sagging from the weight loss. I already told you about the loss of my perky hooters and that I have upper arms with so much loose skin I should be saluted instead of being waved at when people say hi. And we are not even getting to these thighs that look like they need to be starched and ironed.

But at that proverbial end of the day, what matters to me

is that I feel so much better and that I am so much healthier. True, months after the surgery, there were times when I looked at my naked body and broke down and cried. I cried when my breasts fell down. My husband said the sweetest thing to me when they did. He cupped them in his hands and said, "Well, I am glad I was there when the girls were perky." I did not cry merely over the flaws. I cried because I was so small. I missed my zaftig self.

I missed that level of comfort people had come to know, love, and be safe in. I felt safe there, too. I know I have suffered some psychological damage because of all the oohing and ahhing about my weight loss, when I'm thinking that if there's to be any oohing and ahhing, it should be over the fact that I'm telling them I am healthier. What most people seem to care about is that I am smaller. They say, "Girl, you look fabulous." I always thought I looked fabulous. I was a fabulous fat chick. OK, so now people were saying I was a fabulous getting-skinny chick. So why couldn't I just accept the compliment? Why did I see it as a slap at the former fat me? Didn't I say that at my birthday party I was going to have everybody screaming at how fabulous I was? Change is good, but change can leave you a little wacky, too. Oh, yes, I am still a work in progress.

When I feel shaky, I repeat my motto: half the mother, twice the love. No one knows that better than my husband. About eighteen months after my surgery, when I was about one hundred pounds lighter, for the first time in our long years together my husband picked me up. He literally swept me off my feet. I was completely up in his arms, holding on to his neck, and he did not topple over with a hernia or broken back!

"You can probably carry me into the bedroom," I said. He did!

Before: I was taking diabetes medication every time a day dawned, I felt like hell, and I knew I was slowly dying.

After: I must live the diabetes lifestyle for the rest of my life. I still must take an aspirin a day for my heart and Altace, an ACE inhibitor, for my heart and kidneys (down from 10 mg in 2003 to 5 mg in 2006). I have not taken any diabetes medication since July 27, 2003, the day before I had my surgery. To keep it that way, I eat balanced meals, exercise, and test my blood sugar every day to make sure I am keeping it real. And every day—several times a day—I thank GOD for giving me the power to believe that I could do better to manage my diabetes; the power to take drastic action, to reverse the course of a killer disease; and the power to transition from a soul living with the dread of becoming an invalid or dying prematurely to a woman envisioning longevity.

— Food Fit for a Queen —

Healthy meals don't have to be bland and boring. A better diet does not mean giving up all of your favorite dishes. Take mac and cheese. For years, my husband and son never knew that I reduced the amounts of fat and

cholesterol in the dish by using low-fat cheeses, egg substitutes, and either soy milk or lactose-free skim milk.

Here's a sampling of healthy meals my family and
friends have enjoyed at my home.

A BREAKFAST

Omelet Wrap

I fill an eight-inch wheat-flour tortilla shell with a
sauté of green onions, garlic, and sliced turkey, scrambled with Egg Beaters. I season the mix with a few
shakes of Mrs. Dash and a pinch of black pepper. (I
sauté with a butter substitute.)

My portion: about half a wrap, depending on whether
or not I have a few slices of apple, cantaloupe, or other
fruit on the side. I might eat the rest of my wrap a few
hours later.

A LUNCH

Grilled Chicken Cutlet
Salad of Mixed Greens

I usually marinate the chicken in a low-fat Italian
dressing. One of my favorite salad mixes consists of
baby spinach and red-leaf lettuce, with a sprinkling of
chopped pecans or cashews. I often make my own
salad dressing. One is a mixture of freshly squeezed
lemon juice and orange juice, olive oil, minced garlic,

and a dash of hot sauce to give it a little kick.

My portion: chicken cutlet—3 ounces; salad—3 ounces.

A WEEKDAY DINNER

Spicy Tilapia and Veggie Stack
Angel Food Cake with Fresh Strawberries, Blueberries, or
Raspberries

I season the tilapia with a blackened spice or a jerk spice and grill it. I cook a combination of great northern white beans, sliced leeks, and sliced cherry tomatoes in a chicken-based broth. I lay some spinach in aluminum foil, top the spinach with some lemon wedges and tomato chunks, sprinkle on some black pepper, wrap up the packet, and place it on a hot grill for two to six minutes until the spinach is bright green. Dinner is served with the spinach on the bottom; the white beans, leeks, and cherry-tomato combo in the middle; and the fish on top. The dish has everything: protein, vegetables, carbs. And it's low fat!

The cake is absolutely diabetic friendly. I use butter, sugar, and egg substitutes. The cake satisfies the sweet tooth. The fresh fruit blesses the body with needed vitamins and fiber.

My portion: the stack—4 ounces; cake—about the size of a half deck of playing cards; fruit—strawberries, no more than four small ones (sliced), blueberries or raspberries, no more than six.

A SUNDAY DINNER

Five Mushroom Soup
Roasted Whole Chicken
Sautéed Corn
Garlic Flatbread

For the soup, I like a mix of sliced brown button mushrooms, chopped portobellos, sliced cremini, sliced shiitake, and enoki. I drop the mushrooms into chicken broth seasoned with black pepper and a clove or two of garlic. After the mushrooms, I add a little cornstarch for thickening and about two tablespoons of Gravy Master for a nice, rich brown color. I let the mix simmer for about fifteen minutes, then add sliced leeks. Mushrooms have few calories, and their texture satisfies that occasional yen for a piece of beef. Soup is one of the great comfort foods. It always calms and soothes me.

As for the chicken, I season it up real good with my garlic, some Old Bay, and a little Hungarian paprika. Sometimes, I use a Jamaican jerk rub instead. I place a quartered onion inside the chicken's cavity, and put that bird in a 350-degree preheated oven for about an hour and a half or till the juices run clear when I check that thigh meat.

The corn is quick and easy to prepare. In a skillet, I heat a little olive oil. Then I sauté some sliced onions (white or green) and garlic, add the corn and some black pepper, and let that cook about six to eight minutes. Add some sliced tomatoes for color and voilà!

The garlic flatbread is a snap (you can do this in the microwave). Melt some butter substitute, then add granulated garlic. Brush the mix on the flatbread and toast for a hot minute. Sunday dinner is jamming and healthy.

My portion: soup—2 ounces; chicken (with breast meat; my delight)—2 ounces (a roughly 3" x 3" slice); corn—2 ounces. If I want to have a bit of bread, I subtract from the soup, chicken, or corn.

In late summer 2004, my friend Paula M.M. sent me an email about a forthcoming show devoted to diabetes that was in search of hosts with diabetes. She gave me the email address of the show's executive producer, Gary Cohen. I emailed him right away. With all due conviction, I wrote: "Hi, I'm Mother Love. I understand you are looking for me to host your new show." My boldness paid off. He sent me his phone number so we could chat. When *dLifeTV* made its debut in March 2005, I was one of its hosts. I felt blessed to be part of a team increasing public awareness of diabetes, from prevention to optimum management.

As I continue my journey to wellness, many a day I think, *if only.* If only someone had convinced my father when he was twenty-five that he was setting himself up for a short life, I might still have Daddy today, and we could literally be enjoying salad days. If only someone had been able to convince my mother that diabetes was not "just a little sugar," she might have lived to see her great-grandson. If only my sisters Paula and Brenda had not been so cavalier about their health, the former might have lived well beyond sixty, and the latter would not have lost a leg in the fall of 2003, then had heart surgery a year later—and kept smoking! Our sister Marcia, not diagnosed with diabetes, had a heart attack in early 2005, and she was not yet fifty. She also faced the prospect of having knee surgery because of the excessive amount of weight she was carrying. I felt for her. I felt her pain. I felt for her six children, too, thinking how they needed their momma well.

— *Know the ADA* —

If you or someone you love is a diabetic, and you guys are not acquainted with the American Diabetes Association (ADA), make the connection. It's one way to learn more about diabetes, keep abreast of research and new discoveries, learn about meal planning, and get a heads-up about ADA Diabetes Expos and other events in your area, among other things. You can connect with the ADA by visiting its website, www.diabetes.org., or by calling information or checking your local phone book for the ADA chapter nearest you. To contact the ADA by mail, write to: American Diabetes Association, ATTN: National Call Center, 1701 North Beauregard Street, Alexandria, VA 22311. You can also contact the ADA by phone, and the call won't cost you a dime: 1-800-DIABETES (1-800-342-2383). Phone lines are open Monday through Friday, 8:30 a.m. to 8:00 p.m. EST. Live help is standing by. Representatives can provide you with general information on diabetes and refer you to additional sources of information.

It has done my heart good to see my son slowly change his ways: exercising more, drinking less beer, cutting back on carbs. From time to time, I have seen him eating off a small plate, like I do. I pray that Jahmal will continue to keep my struggle in view, along with the prevalence of diabetes in the family; Kennedy's deceased mother was also a diabetic.

I don't have to say a word for Jahmal to get the message: *you can change more easily while you're young and your body is strong. Don't wait until you develop diabetes. Do all you can to prevent getting the disease.* I would never want my son to have to resort to something as drastic as gastric bypass. I say to him and to millions of other people who are battling diabetes and/or obesity: don't do as I did in 2003. Do as I should have done years before then.

If you have an unhealthy relationship with food, especially if you are diabetic, start taking the baby steps to a better diet. Consider thinking about how you came to have bad eating habits. If it's a family tradition, or cultural, recognize that you will not betray your family or your heritage if you pass on eating certain dishes and stop preparing food the way your people have for generations.

Is your problem overeating? If so, ask yourself why. What triggers this behavior? It could be stress in general. Or maybe you are like me, in a family or community where overeating is the norm, and you are going along with the program to get along. Are there some early traumas or deprivations that started you gorging? I have sometimes thought that had I sought out serious therapy when I was younger, I would have been able to stop my overeating before I was at death's door. Again I say, do as I should have done years ago.

— Your Steps to Wellness? —

There is no one-size-fits-all program for diabetics or for nondiabetics seeking to be as healthy as they can be. But there are some basics that everyone should heed. Among them are:

- Get and maintain a positive attitude.

- Do not smoke.

- Reduce your consumption of refined sugar.

- Cut loose heavy drinking—or you may need to abstain from alcohol.

- Do not eat supersize meals.

- If you eat meat, eat lean meat and less meat.

- Eat more fruits and veggies.

- Drink lots of water.

- Reduce your stress level.

- Laugh, laugh, and laugh!

- Get off your butt and move! I don't care if it's swim-ming, walking, or mopping. Just get up and move. Trust me, your hair can handle it!

Think about the possible ripple effect of your journey to wellness! As you improve your diet and eating habits, you could very well influence your loved ones—siblings, parents, spouse, children—to do likewise. You may not bat 1,000, but if your change causes one loved one to kick the bad-diet habit, you've earned your wings. Your change may also prevent others from developing bad habits. Here I think of children especially.

We have a growing number of obese and otherwise unfit children at risk for a host of serious health problems, including diabetes. These youngsters may well become short-lived adults. That does not have to become a reality. We adults must set a better example. Be well.

Lovingly,
The Even More Fabulous!
Mother Love

ACKNOWLEDGMENTS

First I give honor and glory to GOD, who is at the head of my life. To my family, my husband, my friend, my love, Kennedy, you truly love ME! Thick or thin, through *thick* and thin. I love you, baby. He says I am like having a new wife without leaving. My son, Jahmal, who says, "You're my ma; I want you to be well and happy," thank you for my grandchildren who are with us on the planet: Jahmal II, and our sweet baby girl Kennedy, and those who will come. My daughter-in-law, Destiny, I love you with such joy and peace. I am glad we are not just family, we are girlfriends. My sister Paula and my mother, Shirley, who lived with this insidious disease until the complications took their lives, I will miss you forever, and I will fight for my life every day. I love you, I just *can't go out like that.*

My sister Brenda, who has lived with the ravages of type 1 diabetes since she was a child, and the doctors told us she would have no future; I think my niece Sara would have a thing to say about her mommy not having her because of her diabetes! My sister Marcia and my brother Fred know that in spite of what you think of me, I pray for you every day for your well-being, your success, and that of your families. My brother Michael, who is in heaven. My cousin Shelesta, who talks to me, prays with me, and loves me like a sister. Love to all my nieces, nephews, aunts, uncles, cousins, and friends, who may or may not be dealing with diabetes: my auntie Linda and my uncle Andrew, I pray for you to take good care of your health.

To my girlfriends who have been with me since forever—and who, when I started on my quest to better health, did not turn their backs on me like so many others. They believe in me and my mission to heal myself and help others.

> *Lori Smith Lockett*, who still is one of my "Warrior Queens": you always show me there is something new to do in life, with life; we are never too big or too old to dream and make those dreams real. Thank you, Dr. Lori.

> *Derellya Freeman*: you made me do what I never thought I could do or would do—stand-up comedy. You have been with me since the beginning of my

career, never giving up, always willing to work with me even to this day. I love you so much and thank you for believing in me, my talent, my dreams! Where do you have me booked next?

Marti Lewis: you laugh with me, pray with me, love me, and share your family with me. I love you all very much. We are truly sister friends because you'll let me cook in your house.

Paula Mitchell Manning, my first California girlfriend. It does not seem so many years have passed since I moved to Cali, because I was supposed to know you and your husband, Larry. Thank you for teaching me, reaching me, believing in my talent, and being willing to work with me. You are a brilliant writer and we make a great team.

Cynthia Busby: your spirit and light always make me welcome with you whether you come over and are willing to try my culinary concoctions or we are at some swank event you've planned. I am honored to call you my friend.

To the Barker family of Altadena—Roy Sr. and Geraldine (Dad & Mom), Kathy, Bonnie (my California sisters) & Roy Jr.: thank you for allowing us to be in the Barker inner circle, for the words of encouragement, the trips to Cancún, the love, the laughter, and the clubhouse cohorts.

Hiawatha Ware, my hairstylist/girlfriend ever since that day we met on the set of that movie and you said, "I am taking that thing off your head" [my little hairpiece], I knew we would be friends. You are a straight shooter. When I lost all that weight, you made me give up my BIG hair. You showed me I could not carry all that hair with my smaller body and made me fabulous with a new shorter look. You have counseled my new stylist, Kristi Cooke (Headquarters 4 Hair in Pasadena), by phone to tell her what to do with my hair or how to put in a new weave, so she can keep me looking even more fabulous on the West Coast.

An Tran: you are more than my nail tech, you are my girlfriend and I love you. We have some great conversations about love and life. I can come into the shop and just unwind, relax, and get refreshed in body and spirit. Thank you for the love and kindness. One day I will go to Vietnam with you.

My guy friends, you all have been more like brothers to me.

"Uncle" Rudy Spivery: We have known each other since college and can still laugh so hard we cry. We can analyze the situation, any situation, and solve the problems of the world if they would just listen to us.

Mike Yunis, my friend for life! Let it be known now and forever more—Derellya Freeman and Mike

Yunis discovered Mother Love! Mike Yunis put Mother Love on the radio and on the map. I continue to this day to work with Mike Yunis. One day he will quit his job and come and work with me.

Alan Reed: you made living in Cali bearable those first few years we were here away from everybody and everything we knew in Ohio. You made us welcome and let us know we are home here. We have traveled the country and the world together. I always wanted a brother like you. Thank you, my brother. I love you.

Joe Burton: we started out as me, host and you, production assistant and look at us now many years later—very close friends. There aren't too many men I will travel for; you are one. I love you, Joe, because I learned even in this crazy world of show business you can make and have friends, true friends, even if you did leave me in Hollywood for Raleighwood.

Tonya Bolden, writer extraordinaire (did I say that before?), what can I say about you that you don't already know? I would not trust anyone else to put down in words my life stories—the good, the ugly, the really ugly parts—to share with others. This has been the most emotional story, the most costly in my relationships, and I am a stronger, wiser, even more fabulous Mother Love for it. Thank you for all you do for the world! Besides, you know you can peel me like an onion; you make me a better storyteller, you keep me honest and always true to the story. I love you always!

To the beautiful people at Atria Books: my editor, Malaika Adero, who made us cancel all the other scheduled pitch meetings when we went out to sell this story because she knew how much we could do to help heal our communities together. Thank you for seeing the vision. Thank you, Tamara Jeffries, for the awesome work you've done on the resource guide. This has added such valuable information to the book; I know that people will want to keep it at the ready to help them better manage their diabetes. I am just glad I am on the cover!

To the creator of *dLifeTV*, Howard Steinberg. Thank you for the vision and filling the void. To Gary Cohen, Marjan Tehrani, Maria Sandoval, Dori Pitzner, Paula Ford Martin, and the entire staff and board of dLife, thank you for the opportunity to be a part of history-making television and giving the people a way to know we are not alone in our fight. To all the wonderful people who make the TV happen and all our guests who've come and will come to be a part of the dLife family. To my cohosts on *dLifeTV*, For Your Diabetes Life, the talented J. Anthony Brown (you knew it was just a matter of time before we worked together); Jim Turner (I loved your character on *Arliss*; I love you even more); and my girlfriend Miss America 1999, Nicole Johnson Baker, we do work, laugh, plot, and plan well together. I know we were meant to always be friends.

To my American Diabetes Association family: I have been a volunteer with the ADA since my sister Brenda was diagnosed back in the 1970s. I have served in two states, Ohio and California. Thank you to William Rowell, former project manager at the L.A. office of the ADA. He put together the African American Task Force, which I cochair and Dr. Joyce Richey, PhD, chairs. She is also very good at introducing me at events. I love you, Dr. Joyce.

Thank you for all the work the ADA does with the fundraisers, the events, the scientific sessions, the walks, runs, and rides. Peter Knockstead, in special events, thank you for giving the Mother Love Sugar Free Strollers a nationwide presence; thank you to all the staff and volunteers.

Thank you to my physicians, Joseph Pachorek, David Faddis, David Lourie, and Dorothea Spambalg, all in Pasadena. Dr. James Gavin III, thank you for writing the foreword to this book.

I've got to acknowledge my father, Joseph L. Hart. Even though I did not get to grow up with you physically, I grew up with you in my heart. You are always with me, Daddy. I take you with me, your grandchildren know about you, I tell them the stories and show them the photos of you scuba diving, laughing with your family. I think you would be very proud of your great-grandchildren, they are beautiful. I want to keep them healthy. I miss you still . . . I love you always.

To all of my babies, readers, and fans: I love you all so much.

To anyone I missed, thank you, thank you, thank you. Now get this book for everyone you know that deals with diabetes, and that's 20.8 million people. In America alone.

RESOURCE GUIDE

by Tamara Jeffries

$\mathcal{M}$other Love's story is a powerful example of healing. She fearlessly faced her health issues, then took charge and took risks, made tough decisions and tougher lifestyle changes, tapped the strength within and the support around her—all in the name of embracing a healthier way of life. And she did it with humor and faith. She's a wonderful example for all of us. We can learn a great deal from her story, especially if we are facing similar health challenges.

When it comes to health, each person's story is unique. Our genes, gender, environment, health history, diet, activity level, personal habits, health-care options, and the particular combination of our health conditions—as well as countless other factors—impact our health. The very nature of our unique individuality means that when it comes to our health, each of us is on her own path. A treatment that cures one person may not work for another. A doctor who inspires one may turn someone else off completely. Your surgery may be a complete success; mine may result in all kinds of complications.

When we are facing a serious health condition—or even a not-so-serious one—it's good to gather information and support from friends, family members, and other sources. But it's also important to remember that two people may have very similar conditions and seek similar treatment but have opposite outcomes. In other words, your flu ain't like mine.

Perhaps you are reading this book to gain insight into how to handle your diabetes. Perhaps you are looking for the inspiration you need to address your weight issues. You will certainly find both here. But when it's time for you to make decisions about what you should do to address your own health concerns, it's crucial that you make the wisest, most informed decision you can make *for you!*

This resource guide is designed to help you find the information you need to address your own personal health. We hope it can help you understand your condition, locate the right health-care provider, and make informed decisions about your care. Using the information, you can begin to write your own health story—and find your own path to wellness.

Whatever inspiration, insight, or information you find in these pages, however, it's no match for the care and education you'll get from talking to and working with your own health-care provider. (And note: the information here is intentionally general. Your own doctor may have different opinions about what you read in these pages.) It is critical that you get the latest and best information you can from a medical expert. Do your own reading and research—and your own soul-searching, as Mother Love has done—then take that to the best caregiver you can find. Together you can come up with a health plan that is ideal for you.

In Search of a Surgeon

If your desire to lose weight brings you to the sharp point of a bariatric surgeon's scalpel, you want to make sure you're in good hands. It goes without saying that you need to look for the best doctor and the most comprehensive care you can find. But unless you have a medical background, how are you supposed to distinguish a good weight-loss surgeon from a poor one? Start asking questions—and don't stop until you're on intimate terms with your doctor and every aspect of his practice.

Where should you begin? Take a few pointers from the Surgical Review Corporation, a not-for-profit organization that evaluates and selects the American Society of Bariatric Surgeons' "Centers of Excellence." SRC employs a twenty-four-member panel of surgeons and medical experts to review applications from individual surgeons or *bariatric surgery* centers across the country. Those that meet the SRC's criteria for the "excellent" designation go on a searchable list on the organization's website. In order to be on the SRC list, a bariatric surgery center must show that it can do the following:

- Perform at least 125 surgeries a year. (An individual surgeon will have done 125 total, and at least 50 in the preceding year.)

- Provide ongoing education for the surgical staff; make sure the staff is able to recognize signs of surgical complications.

- Have a designated medical director who participates in decision making about the bariatric program.

- Have board-certified surgeons who spend a significant portion of their time specifically on bariatric surgery.

- Have an experienced full-time medical and support staff that can manage the special care bariatric patients need. They should be able to care for critically ill patients.

- Have equipment, instruments, and furnishings that can accommodate severely obese patients.

- Follow standardized approaches to bariatric surgery.

- Have a long-term follow-up program that tracks patients for five years after surgery.

• Provide supervised support groups for patients who have undergone surgery.

How does your surgeon measure up? This is not to imply that only surgeons on the SRC's list are qualified practitioners. Not every surgeon applies for the SRC's designation, so just because you don't find your doctor's name on the list, it doesn't mean he or she is a quack. To determine whether or not your doctor meets your own standards, ask your own tough questions:

• How many surgeries has your surgeon done? Is bariatric surgery his specialty, or does he perform other types of surgery? Find a doctor with lots of experience in the specific type of bariatric surgery you will have.

• What's the procedure like? What can you expect afterward? Your doctor should be able to explain the surgery, possible complications, and expected outcome in terms you understand.

• Ask about his patients' outcomes. Did they have complications? Don't worry so much if they did; that may not be his fault. More important: find out how he handled them.

• Where is the surgery done? Make sure you are at a facility that offers comprehensive care, in case of complications. A bariatric center at your local strip mall may not offer the kind of medical support you may need in an emergency.

• Who is on your team? A typical team might include your surgeon, a psychological counselor, a nutritionist, a bariatric nurse, and perhaps an exercise counselor. How often will you see them? How long will they work with you before *and* after surgery? Is there an additional cost for their services? Because weight-loss surgery has an impact on your body as well as your mind and spirit, you'll want to have experienced people around to help you fully prepare for your procedure and navigate all aspects of your life after surgery.

• How will your doctor help you prepare for surgery? Some programs work with patients for months before they perform the surgery—helping them get as physically healthy as possible and getting them ready for the psychological changes they'll face. You should have a thorough psychological prescreening (possibly several counseling sessions), physical exams, and nutritional counseling. Beware a doc who seems to be rushing you into the operating room. You want someone who wants to understand your health history, lifestyle, and motivations for weight loss.

• Will your team be there for you after the surgery? Look for a program that will give you access to psychological, nutritional, and exercise counseling, as well as thorough medical follow-ups. They should offer or guide you to support groups.

Don't be shy. Talk to people who've had the surgery; check out chat groups to learn about people's experiences with the surgery; and ask about people's experiences with their particular doctors. Don't take their experience as gospel. Use it to help you formulate your own questions.

Do your homework and ask as many questions as you can before you commit to a relationship with a surgeon. It *is* a commitment—and it is a relationship. You'll likely spend weeks or months working with your surgeon and his team to prepare for surgery. And you may return to your doctor over the years for follow-ups. Bariatric surgery is an intimate, emotional process. Make sure your doctor is someone you trust and respect.

Food Factor

When you're dealing with health issues, what and how you eat can make a real difference in your well-being. Food can be medicine—or it can be poison. (Sometimes, it seems, the same food can be both.) And which is which depends on what news report you read; food trends can change almost overnight. Case in point: a few years ago, fat was the bane of a healthy diet; carbs were good for you. Then researchers learned that some fats—like those in fish and avocados—had positive health effects. More recently, eating carbs became a cardinal sin. The nation was back on steak and eggs—hold the toast. But then experts started touting the benefits of whole grains, and toast came off the no-no list.

The lesson: don't get caught up in food trends, especially in those that would have you cut whole categories of food from your diet. When it comes to eating, the important thing is to maintain balance. Eating well-rounded meals in appropriate portion sizes is important to health, no matter your health condition. That said, you may have to modify your diet depending on your particular health status.

People with diabetes, for example, have to be careful not to eat too many foods that will shoot their blood glucose level too high. There was a time when this meant no sugary foods; diabetics had to resort to artificial sweeteners or eat no sweets at all. Today, according to the American Diabetes Association, sweets can be eaten in moderation if they're balanced with the other carbohydrates in your meal. For example, you want something sweet for dessert, you need to skip the rice or rolls. You still have to keep your total sugar/carb intake in check, but, if you play your carbs right, you can have a bite of birthday cake without worrying. Work with your doctor to determine what you can eat—and how much of it—and still maintain healthy blood sugar levels. It may take a bit of mealtime juggling, but it's worth the effort if it allows you to stay healthy and enjoy some of your favorite foods.

Eating plans for people who have had bariatric surgery

are also fairly complex. Even after you've fully healed from a weight-loss surgery, you have a lot to balance. The stomach is smaller, so you're eating much smaller meals; and you may not be able to digest certain foods. At the same time, however, you have to make sure you're getting adequate nutrient intake—which can be more difficult if you've had a bypass operation. Bariatric patients have to be careful and diligent about eating a balanced diet.

If you have surgery, your diet will be personalized by your doctor and nutritionist, but you can expect something like this:

For the first week or two following surgery, you will be on a liquid diet: water, juice, protein drinks, sugar-free gelatin. You'll sip a couple of ounces every half hour or so.

You'll evolve to a pureed diet that may include hot cereal, mashed potatoes, scrambled eggs, thicker soup (but nothing with a lot of fat). Some people eat baby food—which is convenient, though it's probably tastier to puree your own well-cooked food. Doctors advise you to avoid sugary or high-fat foods, which can lead to the dumping syndrome Mother Love describes. You're still eating only two ounces at a time, with two ounces of liquid every half hour in between.

After a few more weeks, you may eat more soft, digestible foods, including chicken, fish, cooked vegetables, and fruits. You'll keep adding foods back to your diet, guided by your doctor, your nutritionist—and your own body wisdom.

But perhaps the biggest adjustment comes after your

body has healed, and you're no longer eating to support recovery. Your body has been altered. The size of your stomach and, depending on what type of surgery you had, the length of your intestine, has changed. But with those physical changes also come changes to the way your hormones work. Your hunger cues and fullness signals may change dramatically. Some postbariatric patients never feel hungry, they say. They have to force themselves to eat. Others find that they have to cope with "head hunger," even though they've eaten and know they're physically full.

Your portions will always be smaller than they were. A typical diet may include only eighteen ounces of solid food per day. That's about a cup of food at a meal or the equivalent of half a sandwich.

Other factors to be aware of:

• You'll need to take a protein supplement for at least four or five months after surgery. Then you have to be careful to get enough of it in your diet forever after. Mother Love's care team suggests that she eat her protein foods before she eats the rest of the meal. That way, if she can't finish what's on her plate, at least she's gotten the protein she needs.

• You'll need to drink between six and eight cups of fluids a day to keep from becoming dehydrated. But you have to be careful to drink in small amounts throughout the day. You can't drink while you are eating. The combination of food and beverage can make you sick. Some say drinking while you eat—or too soon after—can effectively "wash" the food through your system too quickly, which can cause you to overeat.

• You'll have to take a vitamin every day for the rest of your life. If you've had a bypass operation, your body won't be as efficient at absorbing nutrients from the food you eat. Vitamin supplements will be vital to your health; bariatric patients have to make sure they get enough folic acid, iron, calcium, and B vitamins. At first, they'll have to be chewables, because you can't swallow and digest a tablet.

• You'll have to slow down. During the recovery period—and beyond—you'll need to take small bites and chew your food extremely well. Eating a meal will take time, so let your dinner companions know what to expect. And don't plan to eat on the run.

• It may take a while to get back to the food you used to eat. Some doctors say it can take months before you can digest red meat, for example. If something makes you sick when you eat it a month postsurgery, wait a few more weeks, then try it again. If you're fortunate, as Mother Love has been, you will be able to ease your favorite foods back into your diet. But realize that you may not be able to eat certain foods again. Some people can never reincorporate sweets or fried foods into their diet even after they've healed.

The good news is that with careful planning and a little creativity, you can enjoy delicious dining, despite your dietary restrictions. Check out Mother Love's favorite recipes beginning on page 180.

Gain or Lose—Your Weight Is All in Your Head

Whether you are on a diet, contemplating weight-loss surgery, dealing with life after weight loss—or polishing off a box of cookies as you read this—if you are coping with weight issues at all, a significant part of that process is going on in your head.

We tend to think of the process of losing weight as something that happens on a body level. It's about balancing calorie consumption with the amount of exercise we do; finding ways to boost our metabolism; shrinking the stomach, tightening our hips, and singling our double chins. For most of us in weight-loss mode, there's an almost total focus on the body. But, in fact, weight loss begins in the mind, many experts say—because weight *gain* begins in your mind.

Let's break it down. Unless you have the proverbial "gland problem" that is causing your weight to balloon (and most overweight people don't, doctors say), your weight gain comes simply from consuming more calories than you burn—overeating and undermoving.

In order to lose weight, you have to eat less and/or exercise more—a seemingly simple mathematical equation. But the fact is, when it comes to doing that, we have a very hard time. We can't get motivated to exercise, and we have a hard time breaking our consumption habits. The first time we have to go on a diet, we realize that while the key to losing weight may be "just say no," doing so is mentally and emotionally difficult. We're accustomed to eating a certain way. We *like* to eat. And saying no makes us feel deprived. Attempting to lose weight can bring up all sorts of mental and emotional issues.

If you do lose weight, but then gain it back, you may find yourself in a kind of emotional cycle of hope, disappointment, self-doubt, self-blame, and defeat. And even if you lose significant weight and *don't* regain it—as is the case with many bariatric patients—you may find that you have to figure out how to cope with the significant change in your lifestyle, in your relationships, and in your self-image.

How did this cookie get into my hand?

We eat because we have to fuel our bodies. We need nutrients, fats, calories, electrolytes, and other components of food in order to function in a healthy way. Once we've eaten what we need in order to move through the day, theoretically, we should be done with food until we need to refuel.

But we eat for many reasons other than to consume the substances our bodies need. Food eases our boredom, soothes our nerves, and comforts us. We find ourselves eating mindlessly in front of the TV. We reward ourselves after a stressful workday with a rich lasagna dinner and a big slice of layer cake. The image of the depressed woman diving into a carton of ice cream after she breaks up with her boyfriend has become so common as to be a cliché.

Food is often the means through which we connect with the people we care about—so girls' night out often takes place over a meal, drinks, and dessert. The highlight of the family reunion is the huge feast. Food represents love for the mother who cooks all her faraway son's favorite foods whenever he comes home to visit. He eats until he's stuffed, taking in her love in the form of her famous sweet-potato pie.

We also eat because, in our society, it's hard not to. Food is everywhere. We are bombarded with advertisements from restaurants offering fettuccine Alfredo, lobster feasts, baby back ribs, half-pound burgers, and double-meat pizzas. We are convinced we'll be getting "extra value" when we buy our fast food in oversized portions. Even work often centers around eating: breakfast meetings, business lunches, convention banquets, and office parties. Hardly a reception desk exists without a jar of candy for passersby.

The reasons we overeat are many and varied. But when you are trying to lose weight, you have to understand why *you* eat. What pushes your consumption buttons? What food habits have you formed that have become difficult to break? What does food represent for you? What is your emotional connection with food?

Some behaviorists say that we have relationships with food in much the same way we have relationships with the people in our lives. And, just like our relationships with our

friends, lovers, and family members, some of our food relationships are healthy and others aren't. When your connection to food is out of balance or seems to be beyond your
control, that's not a healthy relationship.

Think of it this way: if your spouse or lover is abusing
you, but you can't seem to pull yourself away, you'd recognize that as an emotional problem to be dealt with. If you
can't pull yourself away from food—though your weight and
related health concerns may be threatening your life—you
are dealing with a very similar kind of emotional issue. Until
you recognize, accept, and address the emotional reasons
you're overeating, it may be very difficult to stop doing so.

For this reason, bariatric surgery patients are encouraged
to undergo psychological counseling before their procedure.
The experts have recognized that in order for the surgery to
be successful, a patient has to be able to comply with the
strict postsurgery diet that is necessary for healing, weight
loss, and long-term health. That means you have to change
your eating habits. And, to some extent, the surgery forces
you to. But only to some extent. Experts say that if you work
at it, you can outeat the surgery—a sure formula for regain-
ing your weight.

And if a deep-seated emotional problem is at the core of
your obesity, it's not going to go away just because you've
had surgery. Weight-loss experts tell stories of patients who
were eating because they were depressed. After surgery, they
were still depressed—they just couldn't mask it by eating.
Ideally, this would be a wake-up call to address the underly-

ing issue behind your overeating; in this case, to get at the root of the depression. Unfortunately, in some cases, people find a way to keep stuffing their emotional problems behind food even after surgery—eating constantly, eating nutritionally empty foods, or finding ways to ingest the rich, fatty foods that had been so soothing before. Some estimates say 20 percent or more of bariatric patients regain all their weight. That's not the worst-case scenario. One doctor recalls a patient who, the day she was released from the hospital after her bariatric procedure, couldn't resist eating a donut. She died.

The best weight-loss centers offer a thorough round of mental-health counseling before and after surgery. Precounseling determines whether or not you'll be able to comply with the postsurgery diet and to make the mental changes required to live healthfully after surgery. In the best situations, you will receive counseling until you have sufficiently addressed and healed any underlying psychological issues that feed your need to overeat. After surgery, you'll also get support as you cope with the real, significant changes in your life and lifestyle that obesity surgery will certainly bring.

I've dropped 117 pounds. Now what?

Many people start their weight-loss mantra with, "If I could just lose some of this weight . . ." and end it with some description of a magical new life filled with fun and activity, romance, and career success. People look forward to a new life, and in many ways, they get a new life. When you lose weight—particularly if you experience significant weight loss—you will experience changes. They just may not be the changes you expect.

On the surface, there are physical changes. Yes, you've lost the weight you wanted to lose. But what does your body look like now? Some bariatric patients are disappointed to find that while they've lost significant weight, they still don't qualify as slim. Estimates show that, depending on the kind of obesity surgery you have, you may lose as much as 70 percent of your excess weight. That means you still have 30 percent of your excess weight to lose. And, depending on how heavy you were before surgery, you may still be considered overweight (though you'd definitely be at a healthier weight).

Major, rapid weight loss also leaves many patients with excess skin and tissue that they may not be able to tighten up, even with rigorous exercise. One twenty-seven-year-old patient has said that underneath her clothes she looks like a seventy-year-old woman. Postbariatric patients describe having to wear girdles and sturdy undergarments to hide the excess flab. Some are disappointed to find that, despite their weight loss, they still aren't comfortable wearing shorts, sleeveless tops, or clingy, revealing clothes.

The flab factor can be corrected with cosmetic surgery, but it may require several different procedures—tummy tuck, breast lift, arm recontouring, or a body lift that takes care of thighs, buttocks, stomach, waist, and hips in one procedure. The issue is the cost of cosmetic surgery, which can run into thousands of dollars. In many cases, insurance doesn't cover cosmetic procedures. If you want it, you can expect to pay out of pocket. Fortunately, cosmetic surgery is elective; you don't have to have it. And some people are so grateful for their weight loss and their regained health that they just accept the excess tissue as a badge of honor.

In addition to physical changes are the differences in the way you move in the world—the way you relate to people and the way they relate to you. Some people find that they have more energy and are able to go out and do things they didn't do before. Some people are more comfortable going out to eat; now they don't feel the judgmental stares from other diners. People say they're more willing to go to the movies or take in a show; they can fit into the theater seats. If you're able to join your friends for a bike ride, a game of tennis, a round of golf, or otherwise be more active than you were before, you enjoy the bonus of getting more exercise while you're socializing with others.

But if you're naturally a homebody, or if you've always been shy, your weight loss may not change that. You may be sitting home alone at 150 pounds, just as you were when you were 250. Weight loss changes your weight. It probably will change your health status. But if you want your life to be different, *you* have to make that change.

Some bariatric patients find that their relationships with friends, family members, and colleagues shift as well. Read testimonials from people who have lost weight, and you see that a marriage that was unsteady before one of the partners lost weight continues to suffer afterward. In some cases, a newly thin person develops more confidence and is unwilling to settle for a mediocre relationship. Conflict may arise if a partner is unsupportive before or after surgery. Or jealousy may rear its head in insecure spouses who are afraid the "new you" will be attracted to (or attractive to) a "new someone else."

Friends can get jealous, too. Even if they don't "turn on you," your relationship may change. If you and your buddy were always commiserating about your latest diet efforts, you may find that you don't have as much to talk about once you've lost weight.

Unlike traditional diets, where your weight loss tends to be slow and barely noticeable, bariatric surgery results in a dramatic dropping of pounds. People can't help but notice. And many can't help but comment—about how you look, about how you looked before, about how they feel about weight-loss surgery. Even the most supportive friend or spouse may inadvertently say or do something inappropriate. Their opinions may not be intentionally unkind, but the attention may make you uncomfortable.

But perhaps the most important thing to examine after you've lost a considerable amount of weight is how you think about yourself. Some people have a change in their self-image; dropping the extra pounds makes them emerge like butterflies from old cocoons. Others look in the mirror and don't recognize the person they see there. Still others recognize that reflection all too well: it's the same fat person in a thin person's body. You may not be able to anticipate how you'll respond to your own body until you're standing alone looking at yourself in the mirror. In that moment, you have to be ready to recognize, accept, and move through whatever it is you think, feel, and believe about yourself.

Be prepared for anything. That's where support groups come in. As one patient has said, "Nobody knows what it's like until they go through it." When you can sit and share experiences with other people who have traveled your path—especially those who are farther down the road than you are—you can anticipate situations you may face, gain insight, and get advice on how to handle the changes you'll have to cope with. Postsurgery counseling can also help you deal with such challenges or changes. One-on-one sessions with a counselor may give you an opportunity to work through personal issues that were hidden behind your obesity as well as those that have arisen as a result of your weight loss.

Significant weight loss does have the potential to jump-start a new life that's healthier mentally, physically, and emotionally. It's up to you to take advantage of the opportunity to grow as a person, even as you're shrinking.

In Lay Terms

Here are some terms you may hear as you learn more about obesity, diabetes, or bariatric surgery.

Obesity

bariatrician. A licensed doctor who specializes in treating obesity and its related health conditions. Bariatricians may prescribe diet programs, exercise, lifestyle changes, or medications for weight loss. They do not necessarily perform surgery.

bariatric surgeon. A doctor who is trained and licensed to perform any of several kinds of obesity surgeries.

bariatric surgery. A surgical procedure performed with the goal of causing the patient to lose weight. There are several bariatric surgical procedures: some *restrictive*, some *malabsorptive*, some both. *Gastric bypass* and *stomach stapling* are *not* generic terms for all weight-loss surgeries.

- **vertical banded gastroplasty (VBG).** A surgical procedure that uses bands and staples to create a smaller stomach pouch but does not remove any of the stomach and leaves intestines intact.

• **gastric banding.** A procedure that restricts the size of the stomach by placing a band around a portion of the stomach to create a smaller stomach pouch.

• **laparoscopic gastric banding (Lap-Band).** A gastric banding procedure that is done with a *laparoscope*—a tube inserted into the abdomen that allows the surgeon to view internal organs. A patient has several small incisions in the stomach, rather than one large open incision. The silicone band that is placed around the stomach can be inflated to adjust the size of the stomach as needed.

• **roux-en-Y gastric bypass (RYGBP or RGB).** A procedure that reduces the size of the stomach and also bypasses a portion of the intestine. The more intestine that's bypassed, the less fat your body absorbs.

• **long-limb gastric bypass.** An operation that bypasses an extensive section of the intestine.

• **biliopancreatic diversion (BPD).** A surgery that removes part of the stomach (rather than just stapling it off) and connects the stomach pouch to a point farther down the intestine. Usually recommended for people who are severely obese and need a greater or more rapid weight loss.

body mass index. A formula for indicating your weight status. Using a mathematical formula based on your height and weight, it indicates whether you are underweight, normal, overweight, or obese.

digestion. The process of breaking down food in the body so that its usable components (calories, nutrients, fat) can be used and waste can be eliminated. Most folks think digestion is primarily a stomach function, but important aspects of digestion happen in the intestines as well.

dumping syndrome. Also known as *rapid gastric emptying*, this aftereffect of bariatric surgery causes patients to experience nausea, vomiting, diarrhea, and other symptoms after eating certain foods—especially those that are high in fat or sugars.

intestinal tract. The part of the digestive system between the stomach and the anus. The body absorbs nutrients, fat, and calories through the intestinal walls.

laparoscope. A tube inserted into the abdomen that allows the surgeon to view internal organs without performing open surgery. A *laparoscopy* is a surgery or procedure performed with a laparoscope.

malabsorption. A condition in which the body doesn't absorb nutrients, fat, or calories in the intestine.

metabolism. The process by which your body burns calories, uses nutrients, and generates energy.

morbid obesity. The condition of being more than one hundred pounds over your ideal body weight or having a BMI over 40. (*Ideal weight* is a somewhat questionable and flexible term.)

obese; obesity. The condition of being overweight; having a BMI of 30 or greater.

overweight. The condition of being over your ideal or healthy body weight; having a BMI of 25 or greater.

small intestine. The small bowel; the section of the intestine between the stomach and the colon. Consists of the *duodenum, jejunum, ileum*. The part of the body in which you absorb digested nutrients.

stomach. The pouch, about the size of a football, that lies below the esophagus and above the small intestine.

Diabetes

blood glucose level. Also called fasting blood sugar or blood sugar level. Indicates the amount of sugar in the blood. Diabetic patients regularly test their blood sugar as part of their effort to monitor and control their condition.

glucose. Simple sugar. The body converts carbohydrates, protein, and fats into glucose.

insulin. A hormone secreted by the pancreas that regulates blood glucose (sugar) levels. *Insulin deficiency* or ineffective use of insulin is a cause of diabetes.

insulin shock. Severe *hypoglycemia*. A condition in which your blood sugar level drops so low that you may begin to lose consciousness.

sugar. Any food or substance that turns to sugar in the blood, including carbohydrates, alcohol, artificial sweeteners, natural sweeteners Also: a common term for diabetes in the black community. Instead of saying "I have diabetes," people say, "I have a little 'sugar.'"

type 1 diabetes. Juvenile diabetes; a condition that develops during childhood or adolescence as a result of insulin deficiency.

type 2 diabetes. *Diabetes mellitus* or adult-onset diabetes, a condition in which the body doesn't use insulin effectively.

Sources: American Diabetes Association, American Obesity Association, CDC, NIH National Library of Medicine (NLM): MedlinePlus.

For Your Information: A Resource List

Search the web or check the library, and you'll find a ton of information about diabetes—and two tons about obesity and weight loss. These websites, organizations, books, and programs all aim to offer information and help people better manage their care. Some are offered by medical centers and nonprofit organizations, others by commercial ventures or people with specific agendas. In some cases, the information is based on rigorous research; in others, you're getting an opinion based on someone's personal experience.

When you are working to manage your health—whether it's diabetes, obesity, or another health concern—it's important to do your own research and get as much reliable information as you can. But you can't believe everything you read in a book or on the web. Cross reference information you find, talk to a trusted care provider about it, and use your best judgment when making decisions about your health care.

Below is a sampling of some of the many books, websites, and organizations that offer information about diabetes, obesity, and bariatric surgery.

Books—Weight Loss and Obesity Surgery

A Complete Guide to Obesity Surgery: Everything You Need to Know about Weight Loss Surgery and How to Succeed By Bryan G. Woodward (Trafford Publishing, 2001)

The risks and benefits of weight-loss surgery from an exercise physiologist and nutritionist who develops pre- and post-op programs for bariatric patients.

Gastric Bypass Surgery By Mary P. McGowan, MD, with Jo McGowan Chopra (McGraw-Hill, 2004)

A doctor's-eye-view of gastric bypass, written in an easy-to-read Q&A format.

The Real Skinny on Weight Loss Surgery: An Indispensable Guide to What You Can Really Expect! By Julie M. Janeway, Karen J. Sparks, and Randal S. Baker, MD (Little Victories Press, 2005)

A frank, funny guide by two bariatric patients and their surgeon. Covers the nitty-gritty details of life after surgery.

Winning at Weight Loss By Sherry Torkos (Bearing Marketing Communications, 2002)

A holistic pharmacist and fitness expert, Torkos makes the connection between diabetes and obesity, and gives tips on boosting metabolism, burning fat, and taking supplements to improve weight loss.

Books—Diabetes

American Diabetes Association Complete Guide to Diabetes By American Diabetes Association (Fourth Edition, 2005)

A clearly written manual that defines and explains how to effectively manage diabetes. Includes a glossary, lists of resources, and organizations.

American Diabetes Association Guide to Healthy Restaurant Eating By Hope S. Warshaw (American Diabetes Association, 2005)

User-friendly restaurant nutrition facts for more than five thousand menu items offered by more than sixty chain restaurants.

The Black Health Library Guide to Diabetes: Vital Health Information for African Americans By Walter Lester Henry with Kirk A. Johnson (Kensington Publishing Corporation, 1999)

A comprehensive guide written from the black perspective.

Conquering Diabetes: A Cutting-Edge, Comprehensive Program for Prevention and Treatment By Anne Peters, MD (Hudson Street Press, 2005)

Information on identifying and treating diabetes and prediabetes, includes empowering approaches for managing the disease.

Diabesity: What You Need to Know If Anyone You Care About Suffers from Weight Problems, Pre-Diabetes, or Diabetes By Francine Kaufman, MD (Bantam Trade Paperback, 2006)

Past president of the ADA explains how obesity can lead to diabetes and offers solutions for avoiding the disease, using real-life examples of her patients.

The Diabetes Diet: Dr. Bernstein's Low-Carbohydrate Solution By Richard K. Bernstein (Little, Brown, 2005)

Based on the theory that a low-carbohydrate diet can help people control their blood sugar and manage diabetes.

Diabetes for Dummies By Alan L. Rubin, MD (For Dummies, 2004)

Upbeat but thorough, the guide offers advice on how to deal with diabetes and live a productive life with the "Thriving with Diabetes Lifestyle Plan." Includes useful websites.

Dr. Gavin's Health Guide for African Americans: How to Keep Yourself and Your Children Well By James R. Gavin, MD, PhD (American Diabetes Association, 2004)

President of the Morehouse School of Medicine and chairman of the National Diabetes Education Program (NDEP), Dr. Gavin writes about obesity, diabetes, and other threats to black health.

The Joslin Guide to Diabetes: A Program for Managing Your Treatment By Richard S. Beaser, MD, with Amy P. Campbell (Fireside, 2005)

From the experts at the Harvard-affiliated Joslin Diabetes Center, information about treating diabetes through diet, exercise, and medication; and coping with diabetes in various lifestyle situations.

Reversing Diabetes: Reduce or Even Eliminate Your Dependence on Insulin or Oral Drugs By Julian Whitaker, MD (Warner Books, 2001)

A low-fat, low-protein diet designed to increase sensitivity to insulin and reduce the need for diabetic drugs—with recipes, menus, and exercise information.

Periodicals

Diabetes Forecast

Monthly magazine published by the ADA. Includes information on research and treatment, food and nutrition, stress reduction, exercise, and finding care. Includes an annual resource guide. See www.diabetes.org

Diabetes Health

A monthly magazine that offers information about living with diabetes, including interviews, medical trends, recipes, and charts. There's also an interactive website: www.dia beteshealth.com

Diabetic Cooking

A bimonthly magazine that publishes about fifty recipes per issue—all compatible with diabetic nutritional guidelines but designed to "appeal to the whole family." Also get recipes and articles at www.diabeticcooking.com

See www.mendosa.com for a complete list of diabetes magazines.

Websites

www.beyondchange-obesity.com

A monthly web letter for people who are in weight-management programs, those who've had bariatric surgery, or those who are considering it. Includes advice from professionals and information about obesity treatments, to help people make informed choices.

www.diabeticfoodcritic.com

The site the Diabetic Food Critic ("where diabetics tell diabetics if it tastes good") rates foods marketed and recommended for people with diabetes.

www.eatingdisorderhope.com

Information, links, books, health-care providers, events, and more for compulsive eaters and people with other eating disorders.

www.healthfinder.gov

A service of the National Health Information Center, this site enables you to search for articles and health information categorized by topic, gender, ethnic group, and life stage. Also includes links to hundreds of health organizations.

www.medlineplus.gov

National Library of Medicine website includes a medical encyclopedia, a dictionary of medical terms, and information on drugs, conditions, and treatments.

www.mendosa.com

The personal website of a freelance health writer who aspires "to be America's best writer and consultant about diabetes." Includes dozens of his articles on diabetes, plus charts, links, and reviews.

www.obesityhelp.com

A web support group that offers information about surgery procedures, doctors, hospitals, and insurers as well as a clothing exchange, nutrition-product reviews, chat rooms, and special-interest groups.

www.obesityvote.com

A grassroots program that educates and informs the public about legislative issues involving obesity. Offers tools for communicating with your legislators.

www.renewedreflections.com

Offers information about obesity surgery procedures and life afterward. Includes chat rooms, newsletter, and blog. Best feature: recipes for postbariatric patients.

www.web4health.info

European-based website that answers questions about psychology and lifestyle. Offers many articles on weight loss and obesity.

www.weighyouroptions.com

A campaign of the American Obesity Association, this site defines terms and helps you understand weight-loss surgeries.

Organizations

Advocacy for Patients with Chronic Illness, Inc.

Get free information and advocacy services from a Connecticut-based legal team. Advises on problems with health and disability insurance, employment discrimination, and family and medical leave. www.advocacyforpatients.org

American Association of Diabetes Educators

Professional organization for people who provide diabetes self-management training and information about related conditions. Search the website to find a local diabetes educator. www.aadenet.org

American Diabetes Association

The leading diabetes organization publishes books, distributes information, provides education, and offers support programs for specific groups, including teens, parents, and various ethnic groups. (Special African American initiatives include Diabetes Day and Project POWER, community and church-focused programs.) The ADA call center (1-800-DIABETES) fields 350,000 calls a year. Check the website for links to local chapters. www.diabetes.org

American Dietetic Association

The organization for dietitians, nutritionists, and other food professionals. You can find articles about diet, food, and nutrition on the website: www.eatright.org

American Obesity Association

A political advocacy group, the AOA lobbies to have obesity treated as a disease, improve obesity health care, and address weight discrimination. The website provides information, research, and specific prevention and treatment advice. www.obesity.org

American Society for Bariatric Surgery

A national professional group for surgeons. Check the website to find a doctor in your area, calculate your BMI, or read about the history and description of various surgeries. www.asbs.org

American Society of Bariatric Physicians

Professional organization for doctors who specialize in care of overweight patients and treatment of their related conditions. Search for a physician near you. www.asbp.org

Disease Management Association of America

A nonprofit organization for people who help others manage their health conditions, including diabetes. Search the DMAA directory for information about disease management companies, home health-care companies, and other service providers. www.dmaa.org

Joslin Diabetes Center

Founded in 1898 and affiliated with Harvard Medical School, this is one of the leading diabetes centers. Offers patient care and education as well as conducts research. www.joslin.org

Obesity Action Coalition

Provides education and support to people affected by obesity. Advocates to improve obese patients' access to medical treatments, end the negative stigma associated with obesity, and empower people who are coping with weight issues. www.obesityaction.org

Obesity Law and Advocacy Center

A legal team that assists with obesity discrimination and wrongful-termination cases, and advocates with insurers who deny claims. www.obesitylaw.com

Oldways

A nonprofit food-issues think tank that promotes healthy eating. Order info about the EatWise program, a healthy-diet program based on a Latin American Diet Pyramid. Offers info on food portions, and calorie thermometer to help you manage calorie consumption. www.oldwayspt.org

Shape Up America!

A not-for-profit organization raising awareness about obesity and its related health issues. Provides guidance on weight management, a fitness assessment, nutrition information, and advice for getting active. www.shapeup.org

Structure House

A residential weight-loss facility that focuses on lifestyle and behavioral issues around overeating. Offers a diabetes-specific program, as well as a new program for post-bariatric-surgery patients. www.structurehouse.com

Surgical Review Corporation

An organization that evaluates bariatric surgeons and surgery centers. Search the website for providers in your area. www.surgicalreview.org

Taking Control of Your Diabetes

A not-for-profit group that educates and motivates patients in managing their diabetes and advocating for themselves. Website offers news about products, therapies, and new developments in diabetes. www.tcoyd.org

Weight Control Information Network

Provides the latest science-based information on weight loss, obesity, exercise, and nutrition. www.win.niddk.nih.gov

Other

Diabetes Expo

ADA-sponsored event travels to more than a dozen cities, presenting speakers, info from health providers, exhibits, samples, exercise and cooking demonstrations, and free health screenings. See www.diabetes.org for more information.

dLifeTV

CNBC's program for people living with diabetes and their families. Mother Love hosts with Nicole Johnson Baker, Jim Turner, and J. Anthony Brown. Guests discuss topics ranging from workplace discrimination to sexuality to recipes, and give advice for managing the disease. www.dlife.com

HealthSimple

A company that designs and distributes user-friendly tools for people with diabetes, including flashcards, refrigerator magnets, cheat sheets, and forms. Distributed through the American Diabetes Association's website and the American Association of Diabetes Educators' bookstore.

The Heart of Diabetes

An American Heart Association program designed to educate people with diabetes about the cardiovascular risks. Sign up for educational information, a twelve-week physical-activity program, monthly e-newsletters and daily tips, and a journal to track weight, blood pressure, blood sugar, and cholesterol levels—all free. Email diabetes@heart.org or search the AHA website for more information. www.heart.org

INDEX

Type 1 diabetes, 39, 40–41
  description of, 40–41
  symptoms, 41
  testing, 66
Type 2 diabetes, 40, 41–42, 50, 51,
  66, 84, 113
  in children, 141–42
  description of, 42
  symptoms of, 42
  testing, 66

U

Ulcers, foot, 55
Underweight, 16–17, 20, 30
Urinary stress incontinence, 85
Urinary tract infections, 120
Urination, frequent, 41, 42, 63, 80
Urine, 40
Ursodiol, 134

V

Vaginal dryness, 53
Vaginal yeast infections, 53
Vegetable juices, 119, 132
Vegetables, 11, 69, 127, 136, 188
  healthy, 128–31
  menu suggestions, 181–84
Vietnam War, 46
Viruses, 41
Vision, 53
  blindness, 53, 80, 96, 113
  blurred, 41, 42
  glaucoma, 80
Vitamins and minerals, 28
  daily supplements, 119, 207
  in superfoods, 128–31

W

Walnuts, 131

Water, 119, 120–21, 123, 127,
  188
  lack of, 120
Weaver, Roniece, 137, 138
Websites, resource list of, 227–29
Weight loss, 41, 42, 64, 75
  loose skin and, 87, 117–78, 213–14
  marketing, 162–63
  public reactions to, 133–34,
   161–68, 214–16
  resource guide, 208–16
  saving money and, 169–80
  See also Weight-loss surgery
Weight-loss surgery, 77–94, 109–12,
  117–41
  band vs. bypass, 109–10
  bowel movements and, 134
  diet after, 86, 89, 94, 117–41, 180,
   205–8
  exercise after, 87, 89, 138–39, 180,
   214
  loose skin after, 87, 177–78,
   213–14
  post-op program, 110, 117–41
  resource guide, 208–16
  types of, 89, 94, 109–10, 217–18
Weight Watchers, 73
Welfare, 48–49
Wheat bread, 19
Wilson, August, 133
Women, diabetes rates in, 113
Workout video, 162
Wounds, slow healing of, 42
Wrinkles, 178

Y

Yeast infections, 53
Yogurt, 131, 132

Z

Zinc, 130

242